How to Use This Book

This book serves two different functions. It can either be used as a dictionary of medical genetics or as a concise revision guide/study aid. Readers who already know some medical genetics and require a summary of particular aspects, should consult the contents page. The book is divided into eight chapters each of which contains a number of related topics.

To use the book as a dictionary, look up the word in the Index of Terms (pages vii to x).

Acknowledgements

The author would like to thank Tony Andrews, Ann Chandley, Christine Harrison, David Scott and Tom Strachan for providing illustrations; Lorraine Gaunt and Tom Strachan for helpful comments on drafts.

Index

1 | The Human Genome as DNA

The genome is the total genetic material.

The C-value is the size of a genome (Fig. 1.1). The DNA content of cells is sometimes given as C, 2C, 4C and so on. Normal human cells contain 2C: there are two copies of each chromosome.

Base pairs (bp), kilobases (kb) and megabases (Mb) are the usual units for quantitating DNA. 1μmol of double-stranded DNA is about 600μg or 6×10^{17}bp.

Sense strand is the strand whose sequence corresponds to the mRNA; the complementary strand is the **template strand**.

5′ and 3′ directions. DNA sequences are always written in the $5' \rightarrow 3'$ direction (Fig. 1.2). Quoted gene sequences refer to the sense strand. In the double helix the two strands run in opposite directions. DNA and RNA are always synthesized in the $5' \rightarrow 3'$ direction.

Organism	Size of genome	
E. coli	3×10^6 bp or	3×10^{-15}g
yeast	1×10^7	1×10^{-14}
Drosophila	1×10^8	1×10^{-13}
mouse	3×10^9	3×10^{-12}
human	3×10^9	3×10^{-12}
newt	3×10^{10}	3×10^{-11}
lily	9×10^{10}	1×10^{-10}

Fig. 1.1 Sizes of genomes.

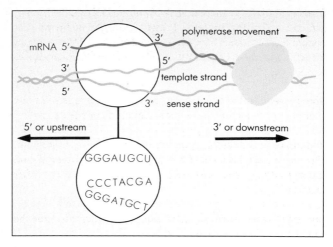

Fig. 1.2 5' and 3' directions in a DNA sequence.

Types of human DNA

A) **Classification by copy number**
unique/low copy number   60–65%
repetitive   35–40%
 	
B) **Classification by function**
protein coding
RNA coding (rRNA, tRNA, 5S RNA)
gene control sequences (initiators and regulators
   of transcription)
chromosomal functions (centromeres, telomeres)
no known function – function undiscovered
                        – non-functional including pseudogenes
 	
C) **Classification by location**
chromosomal genes:
   exons
   introns
   transcription control elements
intergenic DNA
mitochondrial DNA

Fig. 1.3 Types of human DNA.

Classes of DNA. No more than 3–5% of the DNA in the human genome codes for protein. Present evidence suggests that mammalian genomes have evolved untidily with little pressure for economy or neat organization. Most of the DNA appears to have no function.

Unique sequences occur once, or only a few times, in the genome. They include most genes and much other material.

Repetitive sequences are present in many copies per genome. This class includes some genes (e.g. those for ribosomal and transfer RNA, and histones), together with much other material.

Dispersed repeats are identical sequences scattered about the genome.

Tandem repeats are identical sequences clustered together on a chromosome.

Alu sequences are the best known family of human dispersed repetitive sequences. They are good markers of human DNA, e.g. in cell hybrids, because almost any 100kb stretch of human DNA will contain an Alu sequence.

Satellite DNA is the most highly repetitive class. Short sequences are repeated in tandem hundreds of thousands of times. It is mostly located at centromeres of chromosomes, where it may have some role in chromosome function. Some sequences (alphoid satellites) are specific to each chromosome.

Mini-satellites are tandem repeats of, perhaps, 100 copies of some short sequence. There are many different families of mini-satellites, each family comprising one to a few dozen clusters. They have no known function, but are valuable tools for genetic analysis.

VNTR sequences (variable number of tandem repeats) is an alternative name for mini-satellites.

Genes for RNA. Genes for ribosomal RNA, transfer RNA and 5S RNA are organized into tandemly repeated units clustered in nucleolar organizer regions on human chromosomes 13, 14, 15, 21 and 22 (*see* Chapter 2). These genes are transcribed by a specialized RNA polymerase.

Pseudogenes are sequences which are related to functional genes but are incapable of being expressed. At least 10% of sequences detected using cDNA probes turn out to be pseudogenes. They are presumed to be genetic junk with no function. There are two types, processed and non-processed.

Processed pseudogenes appear to be copies of mRNAs. Compared to the parent functional gene, they lack all non-transcribed sequences and introns, but often include a poly-A stretch at the 3′ end. They probably arose by reverse transcription of a mRNA and insertion of the product into the genomic DNA. They are not expressed because they lack promoters, and usually also contain frame-shifts or stop codons.

Non-processed pseudogenes retain the introns found in their functional counterparts. They are not expressed because of mutations affecting sequences such as the promoter or splice sites. They often lie on the chromosome near to related functional genes. The globin pseudogenes are the best-known examples.

The mitochondrial genome. Human mitochondria contain a circular DNA molecule of 16,569bp which codes for some transfer RNAs and some but not all mitochondrial proteins. Mitochondria are transmitted matriclinally, i.e. only through the egg, not through the sperm. There is some interest in variants of mitochondrial DNA, either as a cause of disease or as markers of human evolution.

GENE STRUCTURE

Although the boundaries of the coding sequences can be precisely defined, other less well defined sequences are required to constitute a unit which is transcribed efficiently in the appropriate tissues and at the proper time. These control sequences may lie several kilobases outside the coding region.

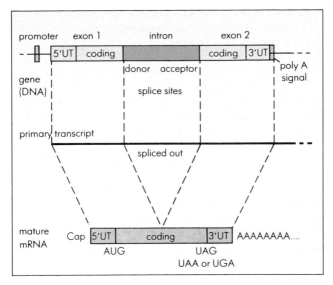

Fig. 1.4 Structure of a gene (not to scale).

Gene	Size (kb)	No. of exons
preproinsulin	1.2	2
HLA Class I antigen	3.5	8
collagen type I	18	52
phenylalanine hydroxylase	100	10
factor VIII	186	26
Duchenne muscular dystrophy	2000	ca.70

Fig. 1.5 Sizes of some human genes.

Exons are the sequences which comprise the mature mRNA.

Introns or intervening sequences are transcribed but then cut out of the transcript during mRNA processing. Wide variation in the number and size of introns is the main reason why human genes vary so much in size. A few genes have no introns. Introns tend to separate a gene into sequences coding for different protein domains or functions, but there is little regularity in their position or number, and none in their size.

GENE EXPRESSION

Producing an active protein product from a gene requires many steps and factors. Failure at any of these stages can cause genetic disease.

Promoters are present at the 5′ end of all genes. They control the start position of the mRNA and govern the general level of transcription. Typical promoters extend over about 100bp and contain several 6–12bp 'motifs' which bind regulatory proteins. An AT-rich motif (the TATA box) controls the start position

Transcription	RNA polymerase II makes the primary transcript using the DNA template. The choice of sequence to be transcribed is controlled by interactions between specific protein factors and DNA sequences near each gene
RNA Processing	capping: addition of a modified nucleotide to the 5′ end splicing: introns are cut out and discarded, and the ends rejoined polyadenylation: addition of typically 200 A's at the AATAAA polyadenylation site at the 3′ end
Translation	ribosomes read the mRNA and assemble the polypeptide, controlled by specific initiation and elongation factors

Modification	may involve:
	    cleavage to remove parts of the chain
	    modification of amino acids
	      e.g. hydroxylation of proline and lysine
	    glycosylation

Transport	within or beyond the cell

Fig. 1.6 Stages in gene expression.

and other upstream promoter elements confer tissue-specific or hormone-dependent expression on the gene. See also HTF islands (below).

Enhancers are short sequences which resemble promoters both in function and DNA sequence, but act at a distance, often of many kilobases. Their precise position or orientation does not affect their function; probably DNA folding brings them into close apposition with the promoter.

Differential splicing. Some developmentally regulated genes produce two or more different transcripts from the same gene by selectively splicing out certain exons along with the introns when the primary transcript is processed. This is unusual; in most genes all exons are always used.

Anti-sense mRNA is synthetic RNA complementary in sequence to a natural mRNA. It can form a double helix with the mRNA which prevents its translation, and so prevents the gene from functioning.

The 5′ untranslated sequence (5′UT) is the stretch between the 5′ end of a mRNA molecule and the AUG at which translation starts. A typical size is 100 nucleotides.

The 3′ untranslated sequence (3′UT) is the stretch of mRNA from the stop codon of the last exon to the polyadenylation site. The 3′UT is often several hundred nucleotides long.

Housekeeping genes code for proteins present in all cell types (e.g. the citric acid cycle enzymes), in contrast to tissue-specific genes such as globin, factor VIII and insulin. The two types may have different promoter structures.

Reverse transcription means making a DNA chain on an RNA template. This is part of the life cycle of many RNA viruses (retroviruses) but is believed not to be part of normal cell metabolism. Reverse transcriptase activity is used as a marker of the presence of retroviruses.

Homeoboxes are thought to be important controllers of differentiation. They were originally found in *Drosophila* as highly conserved 183bp sequences in genes controlling the number and identity of body segments. Humans have at least four, probably a dozen homeoboxes showing 70–90% homology with the *Drosophila* sequences. They are expressed in embryos and appear often to be located near collagen genes.

Transposons or 'jumping genes' are sequences able to excise themselves and reinsert at a different chromosomal position. If they insert into a gene it is usually inactivated. They are recognizable by the inverted repeats which flank them. Human transposons are not well characterized.

DNA METHYLATION

A proportion of the cytosine residues which are in CpG sequences are converted to 5-methyl cytosine by an enzyme which acts only when the complementary strand is already methylated. This perpetuates a heritable pattern of CpG methylation which is believed to be a key signal in gene regulation, in X-chromosome inactivation and probably in imprinting genomes with their parental origin.

Methylcytosine (5-MeC) is lost over an evolutionary time-scale by spontaneous deamination. The frequency of CpG in the human genome is only one quarter that predicted from the bulk base composition (40% G+C).

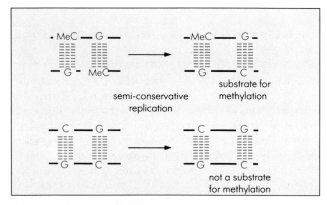

Fig. 1.7 CpG methylation.

8

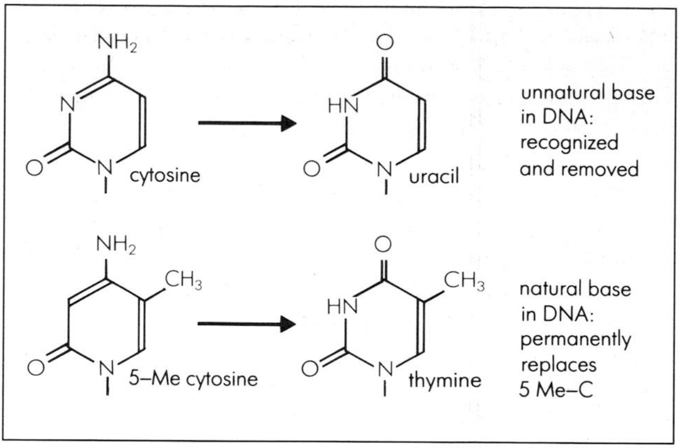

Fig. 1.8 5-MeC is a hotspot for C→T mutation.

HTF islands are regions near the 5' end of genes which are rich in unmethylated CpG. They constitute about 1% of bulk DNA, average 1kb in length and probably have some regulatory role. HTF means Hpa tiny fragments because the restriction enzyme HpaII, which cuts at unmethylated CCGG, makes many cuts within islands. Calculations based on the CpG frequency in bulk and in island DNA suggest that most sites for the enzyme SacII (CCGCGG) lie within HTF islands. Strategies for identifying HTF islands enable the molecular biologist to concentrate on the genes, and ignore the much larger amount of intergenic DNA.

ONCOGENES

Oncogenes are genes whose abnormal expression can transform a cell to a tumour cell. They are conserved across species and their normal function is to control cell growth (Fig. 1.9). Over 30 are known in man. Some encode tyrosine kinases which modulate the activity of target proteins by phosphorylating tyrosines. Trans-membrane tyrosine kinases are growth factor receptors. Other oncogenes encode GTPases which act as second messengers within the cell. Abnormal expression can be due to point mutations, gene amplification or chromosomal translocations. Translocations either produce truncated or

Oncogene	Location	Function	Site of action
erb-B	7p12-p14	epidermal growth factor receptor	transmembrane
fms	5q34	CSF-1 receptor	transmembrane
src	20q12-q13	tyrosine kinase	cytoplasm
mos	8q11-q22	tyrosine kinase	cytoplasm
abl	9q34	tyrosine kinase	cytoplasm
H-ras	11p15	GTPase	cytoplasm
N-ras	1p22	GTPase	cytoplasm
myc	8q24	DNA synthesis	nucleus
myb	6q15-q24	DNA synthesis	nucleus
fos	14q21-q31	DNA synthesis	nucleus
sis	22q12-q13	platelet-derived growth factor	secreted

Fig. 1.9 Cellular oncogenes and their normal function.

fused genes with aberrant responses to control signals, or they place the gene in a chromosomal environment where its expression is inappropriate. Tumour-specific chromosome break points (*see* Chapter 4) often lie near oncogenes.

Viral oncogenes (v-myc, v-fos etc) enable acute transforming retroviruses to transform cells. They consist of a viral promoter fused to part of a gene of cellular origin. Viral activation of oncogenes rarely causes cancer in man.

Proto-oncogenes. The cellular oncogenes were originally called proto-oncogenes and labelled c-myc, c-fos etc.

Anti-oncogenes are genes whose loss leads to neoplasia, e.g. the retinoblastoma gene (*see* Chapter 7). In practice oncogenes and anti-oncogenes are much the same, since both are the sites of mutations leading to cancers.

MUTATIONS

Genes can be changed in many ways, but at the phenotypic level there are changes which abolish the function, those which modify it, and silent changes with no effect.

Region of gene	Mutations likely to:		
	Abolish function	Modify function	Not affect function
Promoter	deletion major change	modify function	
5′ and 3′ UT	remove poly-adenylation signal	change stop codon	other mutations
Code for active site	amino-acid change		silent mutation
Code for rest of protein	deletion frameshift nonsense mutation	non-conservative change	conservative or silent mutation
Introns	remove splice site		other mutations

Fig. 1.10 Mutations and their effects.

Deletion of	Consequences
many genes	*see* chromosomal abnormalities, chapter 4
one whole gene	no gene function
exon material	truncated protein — often unstable; may generate frameshift
intron material only	usually no phenotypic effect
splice site	usually no functional product
promoter	no gene function

Fig. 1.11 Effects of gene deletions.

Deletion is the physical absence of a sequence. Deletions result from non-homologous recombination, from faulty repair of damaged DNA or from a skip during DNA replication.

Insertions are extra sequences, usually transposons or retroviral sequences, inserted into a gene. They usually abolish gene function by disrupting coding sequences, creating frameshifts or interfering with mRNA splicing.

Duplications can be tandem or inverted. Duplication of a whole gene will cause dosage effects only, but partial duplications have the same effects as insertions.

Base substitutions are classified as transitions (A ↔ T and G ↔ C) and transversions (A or T ↔ G or C).

Frameshifts are a consequence of the way the genetic code in the mRNA is read in triplets. Any change in the number of nucleotides in a coding sequence which does not add or remove complete triplets alters the reading frame of all the message downstream of the change. Frameshifts normally abolish the function of the protein.

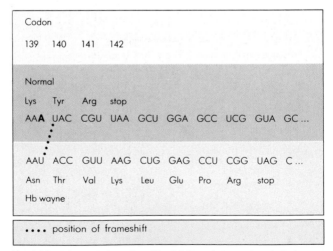

Codon			
139	140	141	142

Normal

Lys	Tyr	Arg	stop						
AA**A**	UAC	CGU	UAA	GCU	GGA	GCC	UCG	GUA	GC ...

AAU	ACC	GUU	AAG	CUG	GAG	CCU	CGG	UAG	C ...
Asn	Thr	Val	Lys	Leu	Glu	Pro	Arg	stop	

Hb wayne

• • • • position of frameshift

Fig. 1.12 A frameshift produced by deletion of one nucleotide (**A**) near the 3′ end of the alpha globin gene.

Silent changes are base substitutions which do not result in amino acid changes e.g. AAA → AAG; both are lysine codons.

Conservative changes are mutations substituting one amino acid with another of the same class (basic/acidic/neutral, hydrophilic/hydrophobic). Any phenotypic effects are small.

Nonsense mutations replace the codon for an amino acid by a stop signal (UGA, UAA, UAG), leading to premature chain termination.

Splice-site mutations alter the 5′ donor (GT) or 3′ acceptor (AG) sequences at the ends of an intron which are required for excision of the intron during mRNA processing. Such changes usually abolish gene function.

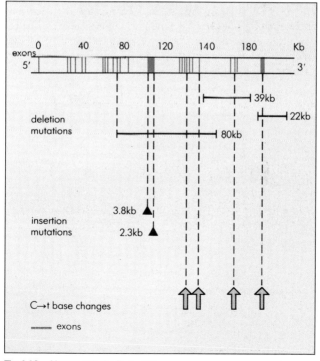

Fig. 1.13 Mutations in the Factor VIII gene.

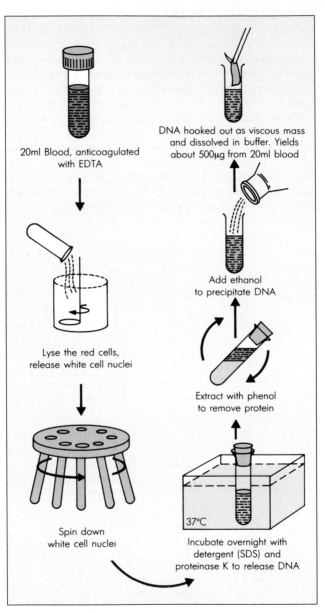

20ml Blood, anticoagulated with EDTA

Lyse the red cells, release white cell nuclei

Spin down white cell nuclei

Incubate overnight with detergent (SDS) and proteinase K to release DNA

37°C

Extract with phenol to remove protein

Add ethanol to precipitate DNA

DNA hooked out as viscous mass and dissolved in buffer. Yields about 500μg from 20ml blood

Fig. 1.14 Extraction of DNA from blood.

DNA extraction usually involves treating cells with detergent and proteinase K to release the DNA, several extractions with phenol to remove protein, and purification by precipitation with ethanol. A great advantage of studying DNA rather than gene products is that for most purposes the type of cell used is irrelevant, since all cells of a person contain the same DNA.

Hybridization means allowing two single-stranded nucleic acids to form a double helix if their base sequences are complementary. DNA–DNA, DNA–RNA and RNA–RNA hybrids can all form. Hybridization can occur despite some degree of mismatch, but the stability of the hybrid is reduced.

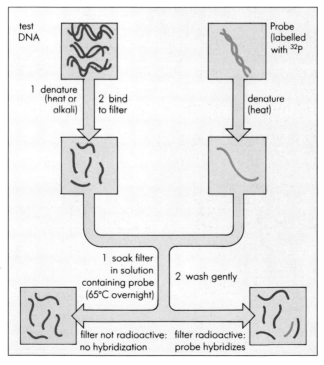

Fig. 1.15 Principle of hybridization test.

Filters in the context of DNA technology are nitrocellulose or nylon membranes to which DNA or RNA binds permanently after baking or UV irradiation. They are used in hybridization tests.

Gel electrophoresis is used to separate DNA fragments by size. In 0.5–1.5% agarose gels at pH 7.5, the migration speed of DNA fragments 100bp–20kb long depends on their length but scarcely at all on their base composition.

Type of probe	Length (bp)	Comments
oligonucleotide	15–50	chemically synthesized
cDNA	100–5,000	cloned in plasmid
genomic (i) random (ii) chromosome-specific (iii) cloned gene	100–40,000	cloned in phage or cosmid

Fig. 1.16 Probes used in human genetic studies.

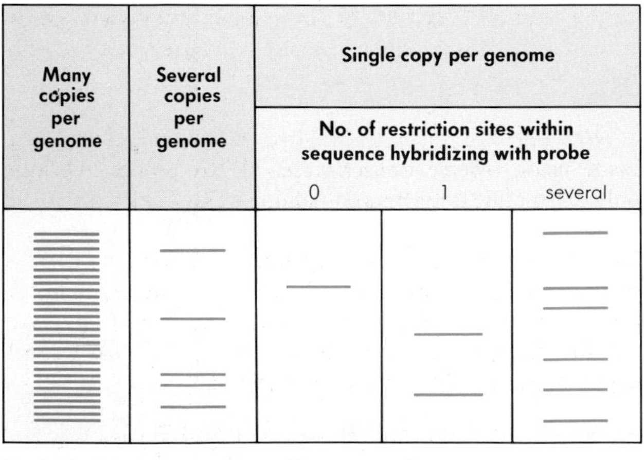

Fig. 1.17 Hybridization patterns with restriction digests.

16

Pulsed-field gel electrophoresis (PFGE) and **field inversion gel electrophoresis (FIGE)** are modifications of agarose gel electrophoresis which can separate DNA fragments in the size range 50kb–10Mb. These size ranges bridge the gap between molecular biology and cytogenetics.

Probes. A probe is any piece of nucleic acid used to test for hybridization. Small probes are often synthesized chemically but most probes are cloned fragments of natural DNA. In order to detect hybridization, probes are labelled either radioactively (^{32}P or ^3H) or with biotin for detection through a biotin-streptavidin system.

Single-copy probes hybridize to a sequence present only once in the genome. Remember however that diploid human cells contain two genomes, so a single-copy probe hybridizes to two fragments per cell (except the X and Y in males). Most clinically useful probes are single-copy.

Repetitive probes hybridize to a sequence present many times in the genome. They are more sensitive than single-copy probes because the target sequence is present at higher concentration. Repetitive Y probes are used for sexing DNA.

Genomic probes are cloned fragments of natural DNA. Most random genomic probes do not include coding sequences, since these make up only a few percent of the total DNA of a cell.

cDNA probes are cloned DNA copies of all or part of a mRNA, made using reverse transcriptase. cDNA probes hybridize only to genomic fragments containing exons of genes.

Libraries are collections of independently cloned fragments. A **genomic library** is made from DNA of the whole genome, a **chromosome-specific library** is made from the DNA of one specific chromosome, a **cDNA library** is made from DNA copies of the mRNA of some specific tissue.

Dot blots are the simplest method of observing hybridization. A solution of the single-stranded target DNA is spotted onto a filter for hybridization testing. (*See* p.22).

In situ hybridization means bathing a suitably prepared tissue section or chromosome spread in labelled probe in order to see which cells or chromosomes bind the probe. In situ hybridization of a probe to mRNA is used to study spatial and temporal patterns of gene expression. Probes for in situ hybridization are labelled with tritium or by a non-radioactive method, rather than with ^{32}P.

Gene amplification is used to increase the proportion of a sequence of interest against a background of irrelevant DNA. In theory each cycle of the **polymerase chain reaction** (PCR) doubles the desired sequence without increasing the unwanted

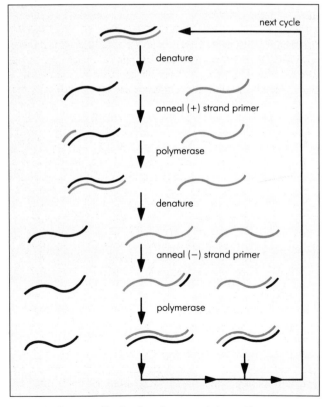

next cycle

denature

anneal (+) strand primer

polymerase

denature

anneal (−) strand primer

polymerase

Fig. 1.18 Gene amplification by polymerase chain reaction.

sequences. In practice 30 cycles give 10^5–10^6 fold amplification. Single copy human sequences become detectable by much simplified methods after amplification. The primers must specifically hybridize on either side of the sequence to be amplified, so PCR can be used only for genes whose sequence is known, so that suitable primers can be designed.

The term gene amplification is also used to describe a naturally-occurring amplification of certain genes seen either as a normal developmental process (e.g. ribosomal RNA genes amplified in amphibian oocytes) or in abnormal cells produced by strong selection (e.g. methotrexate-resistant cell lines usually have the dihydrofolate reductase gene amplified).

RESTRICTION ENZYMES

Restriction enzymes are endonucleases which cut double-stranded DNA only at a certain specific sequence (the recognition or restriction site). Over 200 are known, each with its particular recognition site. These are usually palindromic 4 or

Enzyme	Source	Sequence cut	Average fragment size Kb
HaeIII	*Haemophilus aegyptus*	GGCC	0.6
TaqI	*Thermus aquaticus*	TCGA	1.1
MspI	*Moraxella* species	CCGG	2.5
HpaII	*Haemophilus parainfluenzae*	CCGG	2.5
HinfI	*Haemophilus influenzae* Rf	GANTC	0.3
EcoRI	*Escherichia coli* R factor	GAATTC	3.0
HindIII	*Haemophilus influenzae* Rd	AAGCTT	3.0
PstI	*Providencia stuartii*	CTGCAG	7.0
BamHI	*Bacillus amyloliquefaciens* H	GGATCC	7.0
SmaI	*Serratia marescens*	CCCGGG	62.5
SacII	*Streptomyces achromogenes*	CCGCGG	250
MstII	*Microcoleus* species	CCTNAGG	7.0
NotI	*Norcadia otitidis-caviarum*	GCGGCCGC	6250

*assuming 40% G+C but only 25% of the predicted CpG

Fig. 1.19 Restriction enzymes. N means any nucleotide.

19

6bp sequences (i.e. each strand, read in the 5′–3′ direction, is the same).

4-cutters are restriction enzymes with a 4-base recognition site.

6-cutters are restriction enzymes with 6-base recognition sites, which usually give larger fragments than 4-cutters.

Rare-cutters are enzymes such as NotI or SacII whose recognition sites occur infrequently, because they are large, contain

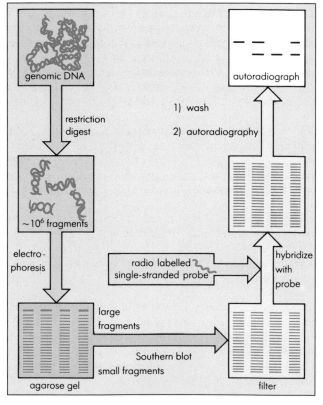

Fig. 1.20 Southern blotting.

CpG's, or both. These enzymes are important tools for long-range mapping (*see* Chapter 3).

Methylation-sensitive enzymes have a recognition site including –CpG–, which must be unmethylated. HpaII is methylation sensitive but MspI is not; differences in the way they cut DNA show where it is methylated.

Restriction digests are made by incubating DNA with a restriction enzyme until every site for that enzyme has been cut. A typical 6-cutter would cleave the human genome into 1 million fragments. Digests used in human mapping or diagnosis typically contain the DNA of about 10^6 cells ($5\mu g$).

Restriction analysis means studying the sizes of fragments in a restriction digest by gel electrophoresis. For simple mixtures (viral or plasmid genomes, or amplified human DNA) the fragments can be visualized directly as UV fluorescent bands in gels stained with ethidium bromide. Unamplified human DNA gives an unresolvable smear; individual fragments are visualized by hybridization to a labelled probe.

Southern blotting is a method of transferring undisturbed a pattern of DNA fragments from an agarose gel onto a filter, where they can be tested for hybridization. This is the most common form of DNA study performed for clinical genetic purposes. The name comes from the inventor, Dr EM Southern.

Northern blotting is the transfer of RNA fragments from a gel to a filter, analogous to the Southern blot.

Western blotting is the transfer of proteins from electrophoretic gel to nitrocellulose filters.

Locus-specific probes hybridize to only one particular gene, but are not sensitive to minor variations in the target sequence, such as often distinguish different alleles of a gene. DNA hybridization does not require a perfect match, and if a probe is a few hundred bases long, hybridization is not prevented by a few mismatched base pairs.

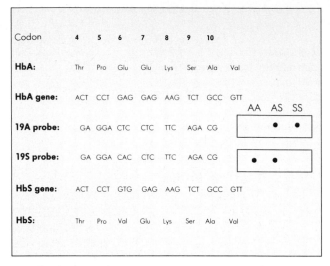

Fig. 1.21 Diagnosis of sickle-cell disease using allele-specific probes in dot blots.

Allele-specific probes are oligonucleotides often chosen to be about 20 bases long, whose hybridization with the target sequence (in carefully controlled conditions) is upset by a single base-pair mismatch. They are best used after amplifying the target sequence. Allele-specific probes can be used to test a DNA sample for the presence or absence of a particular mutation. Their disadvantage is that they detect only that specific mutation, not any mutated version of the gene. Thus they are not appropriate for the many human diseases which are heterogeneous at the DNA level.

RESTRICTION FRAGMENT LENGTH POLYMORPHISMS

Restriction Fragment Length Polymorphisms (RFLPs) are inherited differences between the DNA of normal healthy people revealed by Southern restriction analysis. With most probes and enzymes, different people give the same band pattern. The pattern of bands seen on the autoradiogram depends on the choice of probe.

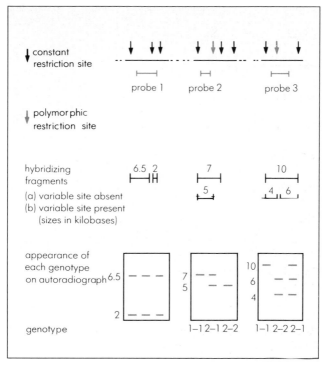

Fig. 1.22 Restriction analysis using 3 different probes.

Occasionally the DNA fragment hybridizing with the probe is a different length in different people, or in the two chromosomes present in one person. There are two possible reasons for this:

- about 1 nucleotide in 150 is polymorphic. If a polymorphic variant creates or abolishes a restriction site it will change the pattern of fragments produced in a restriction digest.
- two constant restriction sites may be a different distance apart in different people if lying between them is a VNTR sequence. Tandemly-repeated DNA elements are particularly likely to vary in copy number between people because the copy number can change by unequal recombination (*see* Chapter 2).

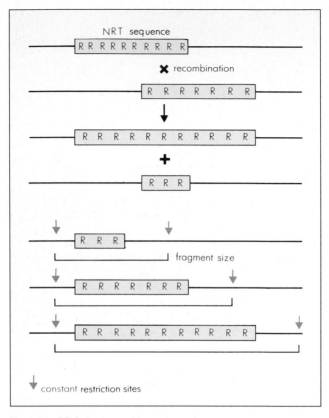

Fig. 1.23 RFLP due to variable numbers of tandem repeats.

DNA fingerprints are made by hybridizing a mini-satellite probe to a Southern blot of restriction fragments. Each band corresponds to one tandemly repeated cluster; the different clusters in one person have different copy numbers, so they give different size bands. The pattern from a person's DNA constitutes a unique genetic fingerprint, specific to that individual (except for identical twins). In Fig. 1.24 the twins in tracks 2 and 3 are monozygotic but those in tracks 4 and 5 are dizygotic. Each band is inherited from one parent and therefore fingerprints can be used for paternity testing (compare tracks 1, 6, 7 and 8 in Fig. 1.24.

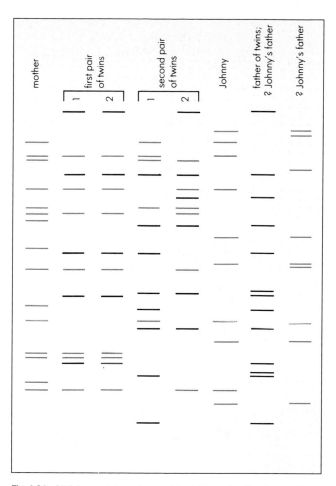

Fig. 1.24 DNA fingerprinting using a mini-satellite probe. Bands are colour coded to show their parental origin.

2 | The Human Genome as Chromosomes

In all cells DNA is organized into **chromosomes**. These usually exist as extended 30nm fibres, too thin to see under the light microscope. When a cell divides, the DNA forms compact bundles which are genetically inactive but visible under the microscope. Chromosomal organization on a scale visible under the light microscope is largely irrelevant to the coding function of the DNA, but it governs the transmission of DNA from generation to generation.

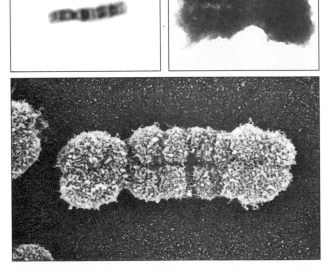

Fig. 2.1 A mitotic chromosome: (a) light microscope, (b) scanning em and (c) transmission em.

Chromatids. As seen in mitosis, each chromosome consists of two chromatids. This is not however the normal state of a chromosome in the cell. During interphase and G1 phase of the cell cycle there is only a single chromatid. Only cells which are committed to mitosis enter S phase, when the DNA is replicated, forming two identical **sister chromatids**. After mitosis, each daughter cell again has only a single chromatid.

STRUCTURE OF CHROMOSOMES

A diploid human cell contains about 2 metres of DNA. It is organized on at least three levels: nucleosomes, the 30nm fibre, and the loop-and-scaffold structure of chromosomes.

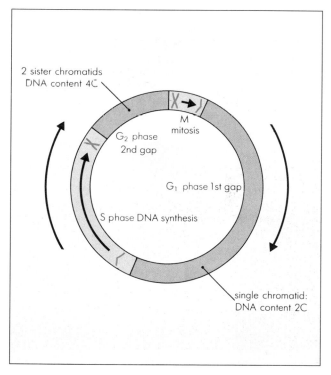

Fig. 2.2 The chromosome during the cell cycle.

Nucleosomes are complexes of eight histone molecules, two each of H2A, H2B, H3 and H4. Round each complex is wrapped 146bp of DNA with 20–100bp free between adjacent nucleosomes. The DNA in the interphase cell as well as in the visible chromosomes is assumed to exist in this form.

The 30nm fibre is the basic unit of chromatin, comprising strings of nucleosomes associated with histone H1 and other proteins, and coiled in some way.

Central scaffold forming the axis of chromosomes consists mainly of two proteins, Sc1 and Sc2. Sc1 may be an enzyme with DNA cutting and joining activity which regulates super-coiling of DNA (a topoisomerase). The scaffold is thought to exist both in interphase and metaphase chromosomes.

Chromatin loops varying in size are believed to radiate from the scaffold. Each loop may perhaps represent a single tran-scription unit or regulated domain.

Ploidy means the number of copies of the genome which a cell contains.

Homologous chromosomes. Diploid cells have two copies of each chromosome (except the X and Y in males). The pairs, such as the two number 1's, are called homologues. Homo-logues are not exact duplicates; they come from different parents. They are similar in that each carries the same genetic loci, but they are different in that, for example, at the ABO blood group locus on chromosome 9, one number 9 might carry the allele for group A and its homologue might carry the allele for group O.

Chromatin is the non-specific name for the material out of which chromosomes are made. It contains DNA, histones and a variety of non-histone proteins which package the DNA and regulate its activity.

Heterochromatin is more tightly condensed and in cytological preparations stains darker than the remaining material (**euchromatin**). It is particularly found at centromeres and on the Y chromosome, and is believed to be genetically inactive.

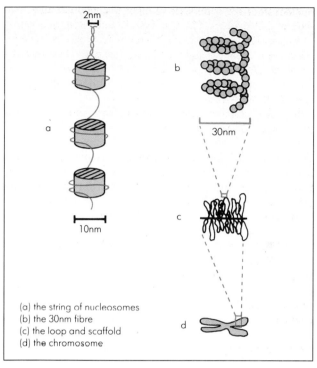

(a) the string of nucleosomes
(b) the 30nm fibre
(c) the loop and scaffold
(d) the chromosome

Fig. 2.3 Structure of chromosomes.

Ploidy	DNA content	No of chromosomes	Cell type
Haploid	C	23	Sperm, egg pronucleus
Diploid	2C	46	All normal somatic cells
Triploid	3C	69	Abnormal cells only (Ch. 4)
Tetraploid	4C	92	Some liver cells etc.

Fig. 2.4 Ploidy of human cells.

Interphase chromosome configuration is studied by in situ hybridization with chromosome-specific DNA probes labelled with fluorescent or other microscopically visible chemicals. This 'chromosome painting' enables individual chromosomes and some gross structural changes to be recognized in the interphase nucleus and sites of attachment to the nuclear membrane to be discerned.

Three levels of duality. A diploid cell has two homologous copies of each chromosome. Each of the homologues, as seen in mitotic preparations, has two sister chromatids. Each chromatin has the genetic material as a double DNA helix. Nevertheless there are only two copies of each gene in the cell, not eight. Only one strand of the double helix acts as a template for transcription, and normal cells (i.e. cells of G1 phase of the cell cycle) have only one chromatid of each homologue.

CELL DIVISION

Cell cycle genes govern the invisible biochemical changes which commit a cell in G_1 phase to DNA synthesis and eventual cell division, and which allow a G_2 cell to proceed to mitosis. They have mainly been identified in yeast, but human homologues have been found for some yeast cell cycle genes. The proto-oncogene c-myc (*see* Chapter 1) is probably a cell cycle gene.

Mitosis	Meiosis
Produces somatic cells	Produces gametes
Daughter cells are genetically identical	Daughter cells are genetically different
Daughter cells diploid (46 chromosomes)	Daughter cells haploid (23 chromosomes)

Fig. 2.5 Mitosis and meiosis: the results.

Mitosis is the normal process of cell division. During mitosis one sister chromatid of each chromosome is passed to each daughter cell. Sister chromatids are exact copies of one another, as far as the fidelity of DNA replication allows, therefore the daughter cells are genetically identical. All the cells of an adult's body, except sperm or egg cells, are derived by repeated mitosis from the original fertilized egg. In mitosis each chromosome behaves independently. Homologues do not show any particular relationship to one another in a metaphase spread such as Fig. 2.13; the only non-random arrangement in human mitosis is a tendency of the satellites which are seen on variable numbers of copies of chromosomes 13–15, 21 and 22 to lie together (satellite association). Because chromosomes behave independently in mitosis, mitosis (unlike meiosis) proceeds normally in cells with abnormal ploidy and in cells with chromosomal rearrangements such as translocations. Recombination does occur in mitosis, but at very low frequency compared to meiosis; an example of mitotic recombination is shown in Fig. 7.12.

Meiosis is the specialized cell division which produces gametes (sperm and egg). Its function is to make gametes haploid and genetically different.

Mitosis	Meiosis
Seen in all tissues	Seen only in testis and ovary
1 round of DNA replication 1 round of cell division	1 round of DNA replication 2 rounds of cell division
Simple prophase	Long complex prophase I
Homologues behave independently	Homologous chromosomes pair
Recombination rare and abnormal	Recombination is normal

Fig. 2.6 Mitosis and meiosis: the mechanism.

Interphase. Nucleus bounded by membrane. No chromosomes visible.

Prophase. The submicroscopic chromatin threads gradually contract until the individual chromosomes are visible.

Metaphase. Nuclear membrane dissolves. 46 chromosomes, each comprising two sister chromatids joined at the centromere, are distributed over the metaphase plate. Chromosomes maximally contracted.

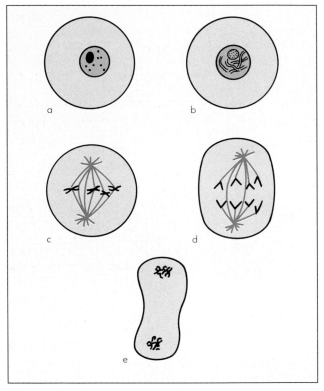

Fig. 2.7 Stages of mitosis: (a) interphase, (b) prophase, (c) metaphase, (d) anaphase and (e) telophase.

Anaphase. Each centromere splits. One chromatid of each chromosome is pulled to each pole of the cell by spindle fibres attached to the centromere.

Telophase. Chromatids reach pole and start to de-condense. Nuclear membranes re-form. Cytoplasm starts to divide (cytokinesis).

MEIOSIS

There are two divisions. In males the product is four spermatozoa; in females the cytoplasm divides unequally at each stage, giving the oocyte and the first and second polar bodies.

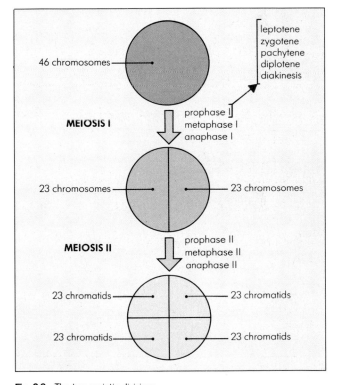

Fig. 2.8 The two meiotic divisions.

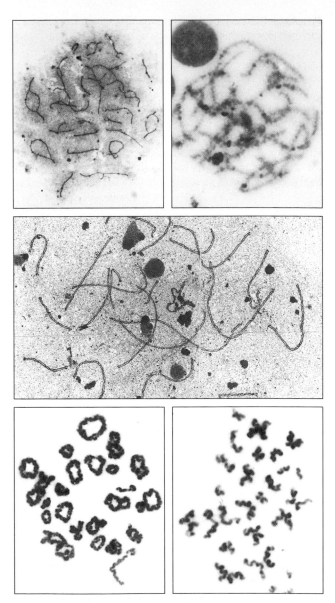

Fig. 2.9 Stages of meiosis: (a) zygotene, (b) late pachytene, (c) pachytene (em), (d) metaphase I and (e) metaphase II.

Prophase I is divided into leptotene, zygotene, pachytene, diplotene and diakinesis.

Leptotene chromosomes are unpaired fine threads each consisting of two tightly bound sister chromatids.

Zygotene is the stage when homologues pair to form bivalents. The threads are still extremely fine.

Pachytene chromosomes are thicker and countable. Under the electron microscope the paired homologues are clear. Crossing over occurs at this stage.

Diplotene bivalents take on characteristic shapes as the homologues separate but are held together by chiasmata. Crossovers can be counted and their positions logged.

Diakinesis is the last stage of prophase I, with the bivalents more contracted.

Metaphase I is reached when the nuclear membrane dissolves. Pairs of homologous two-stranded chromosomes are held together by chiasmata.

Anaphase I. In contrast to mitosis, centromeres do not split. One complete two-stranded chromosome from each bivalent goes to each pole.

Meiosis II resembles mitosis. Centromeres split at metaphase II and single chromatids move to the poles.

RECOMBINATION

During prophase I of meiosis homologous chromosomes are cut and rejoined so as to exchange segments.

Bivalents are the four-stranded structures comprising paired two-stranded homologues which form at zygotene and dissolve at metaphase I. At diplotene and later their shape is dictated by the number of chiasmata.

Chiasmata or **crossovers** are the exchanges between homologues within a bivalent, which are seen in diplotene, diakinesis and metaphase I of meiosis. Each crossover involves two of the four chromatids, so that double recombinants may involve two, three or all four strands. In human male meiosis an average of 55 chiasmata are seen with at least one in each bivalent. The chiasma count is higher in female meiosis.

Synapsis is the intimate pairing of homologous chromosomes in zygotene and pachytene of meiosis, which is a prerequisite for crossing over. Synapsis uses an unknown mechanism (un-

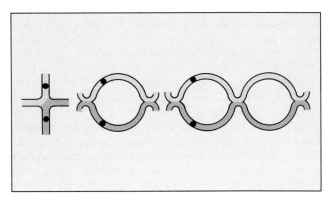

Fig. 2.10   Bivalents with 1, 2 and 3 chiasmata.

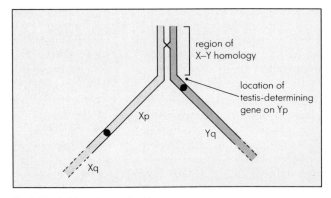

Fig. 2.11   X–Y homology and pairing.

likely to be Watson–Crick base pairing) to align matching sequences. If a chromosome has a section rearranged relative to its homologue, the bivalent usually forms so that matching sequences synapse.

The synaptonemal complex is a protein structure which appears to hold together the two homologous chromosomes in pachytene bivalents.

X–Y pairing and homology. In male meiosis the X and Y pair by the tips of the short arms (Fig. 2.11). These regions, but not the rest of the chromosomes, are homologous and one obligatory crossover takes place in this restricted region. The few genes located in this region show pseudo-autosomal inheritance.

CHROMOSOME PREPARATION

As a source material, spontaneously dividing cells are present only in bone marrow, trophoblast, and testis . The other tissues must be grown in culture to obtain dividing cells. Culture times vary from 48 hours for blood to 1–3 weeks for amniotic fluid. Even tissues with spontaneously dividing cells are often cultured briefly (short term culture) to improve the mitotic index. Blood is the most convenient material for mitotic studies because it is easily obtained, culture times are short and good quality preparations are easily obtained.

Source	Cell	Application
blood	T-lymphocytes	routine analysis
skin	fibroblasts	suspected mosaics
bone marrow	white cells etc	leukaemia
amniotic fluid	shed epithelium	16–20wk fetus
chorionic villi	trophoblast	8–14wk fetus
buccal smear	shed epithelium	sex chromatin
testicular biopsy	spermatocytes	male meiosis
fetal ovary	oocytes	female meiosis
sperm	spermatozoa	male meiosis

Fig. 2.12 Materials for chromosome study.

The aim of chromosome preparation is to produce a good yield of cells with well-spread chromosomes. A typical protocol would be:

- a population of rapidly growing cells is obtained
- colchicine or colcemid is added to increase the mitotic index
- cells are suspended in hypotonic saline. This makes them swell and separates the chromosomes, which otherwise tend to form tangled masses
- cells are fixed and spread on microscope slides
- the chromosomes are stained, either homogeneously or with banding.

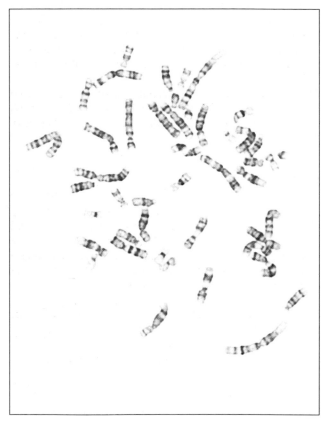

Fig. 2.13 A spread suitable for chromosome analysis.

The mitotic index is the proportion of cells which are in mitosis when the specimen is examined.

Colchicine and its synthetic derivative colcemid disrupt the spindle fibres which pull chromatids apart at anaphase. Colchicine-treated cultures accumulate cells in metaphase.

Synchronized cultures have all cells reaching mitosis at the same predictable time. This makes it possible to catch cells in late prophase for high-resolution banding. DNA replication is blocked with methotrexate or excess thymidine; cells accumulate in S-phase and all move forward together when the block is released.

Phytohaemagglutinin (PHA) is a plant lectin which stimulates T-lymphocytes to divide. PHA stimulation enables blood cultures to be grown up for chromosome analysis in only 48 hours.

Sperm chromosomes can be studied by allowing spermatozoa to penetrate hamster eggs which have been stripped of the zona pellucida. Inside the egg, the tightly packed chromosomes of the sperm spread out.

THE NORMAL KARYOTYPE

The karyotype is the chromosome constitution of a cell, e.g. 46,XY. The term is also often used for figures which should strictly be called Karyograms. Karyograms are prepared from photographs by cutting up the print and shuffling chromosomes around, or by the equivalent procedure in an image analysis computer.

Sex chromosomes are the X and Y chromosomes. Normal females are 46,XX and normal males 46,XY.

Autosomes are all the chromosomes except the X and Y.

Unbanded karyotype. Uniformly stained (unbanded) chromosomes are classified into seven groups. Some can be recognized individually, but the C group chromosomes in particular cannot all be paired up with any confidence.

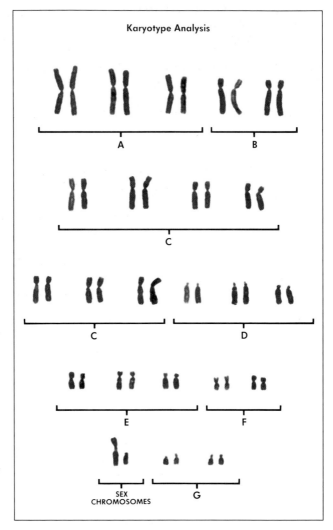

Fig. 2.14 Unbanded karyotype.

The centromere or **kinetochore** is the point at which sister chromatids are joined, and the attachment point for spindle fibres during cell division. The centromere splits at metaphase of mitosis and metaphase II of meiosis.

The **centromeric index** is the distance of the centromere from the tip of the short arm, expressed as a percentage of total chromosome length.

Metacentric chromosomes have the centromere roughly in the middle, e.g. human chromosomes 1, 3, 16, 19 and 20.

Submetacentric chromosomes have the centromeric index in the range 20–40, e.g. human chromosomes 2, 4–12, 17, 18 and X.

Acrocentric chromosomes have the centromere close to one end, as in human chromosomes 13–15, 21, 22 and Y.

Telocentric chromosomes have the centromere right at the end. Humans have no telocentric chromosomes.

Group	Chromosomes	Description
A	1–3	largest, metacentric to submetacentric
B	4, 5	large, arms very unequal
C	6–12, X	medium size, submetacentric
D	13–15	medium size, acrocentric
E	16–18	small, metacentric or submetacentric
F	19, 20	small, metacentric
G	21, 22, Y	small, acrocentric

Fig. 2.15 Human chromosome groups.

Acentric chromosomes are abnormal chromosomes lacking a centromere. They do not attach to the spindle and are often lost at cell division by anaphase lag.

Dicentric chromosomes are abnormal chromosomes with two centromeres. Unless the two are very close together, they risk being pulled in opposite directions at anaphase, leading to anaphase lag or chromosome breakage.

Telomeres are the ends of chromosomes. They contain special DNA sequences essential to chromosome stability. Ends without telomeres, created by breakage, are rejoined by cellular repair mechanisms; faulty repair of broken ends is a common cause of structural chromosome abnormalities.

Satellites are small knobs on stalks projecting from the short arms of some copies of chromosomes 13, 14, 15, 21 and 22. They vary in size and number between normal individuals.

Satellite association is the tendency for satellited chromosomes to lie close to each other in mitotic spreads.

CHROMOSOME BANDING

A variety of disruptive treatments cause chromosomes to stain in reproducible patterns of dark and light bands. The development of banding (Caspersson 1968) was a seminal advance in cytogenetic technique, enabling each chromosome to be identified individually for the first time.

G-banding: chromosomes are subjected to a controlled digestion with trypsin then stained with Giemsa. This is the standard banding method in most laboratories. The differential staining reflects differences in the DNA. Pale G-bands are relatively rich in A+T, in genes and in Alu sequences (see Chapter 1). Dark G-bands are G + C rich, poorer in genes, and contain a different class of repetitive DNA element, the LINE sequence. Regions which stain as dark G-bands show as grooves in the scanning electron microscope (see Fig. 2.1b).

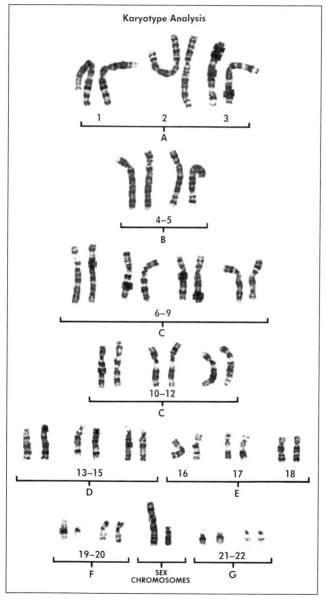

Fig. 2.16 G-banded karyotype.

43

High resolution banding means studying chromosomes in late prophase (prometaphase) when they are not fully contracted. The 400 G-bands seen in metaphase preparations split into 850 or more sub-bands. The more extended chromosomes are harder to disentangle and identify, but smaller abnormalities can be seen. Even at the highest resolution (3000 bands) the average band contains 1 megabase of DNA.

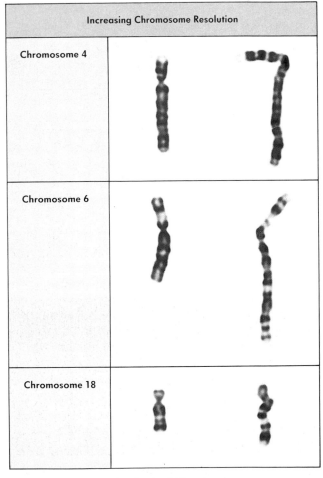

Fig. 2.17 High-resolution banding (partial karyotypes).

C-banding stains centromeres plus certain other heterochromatic regions. This is useful for suspected dicentric or acentric chromosomes. C-banding is produced by treatment with barium hyroxide and staining with Giemsa.

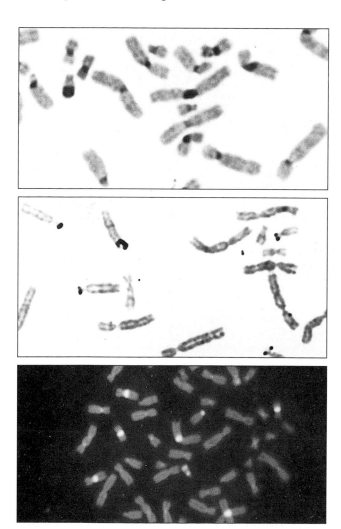

Fig. 2.18 Examples of: (a) C-banding, (b) silver staining and (c) distamycin-DAP1 fluorescence.

Fluorescence staining uses dyes which make certain regions fluoresce in UV light e.g. distamycin A + DAPI (4, 6-diamidino 2-phenyl indole) give brilliant fluorescence in the heterochromatic regions of chromosomes 1, 9, 16 and Y, plus the short arm of chromosome 15.

Q-banding uses the ultraviolet fluorescence of chromosomes stained with quinacrine. The pattern is mostly the same as G-banding. The long arm of the Y chromosome fluoresces intensely and even in non-dividing cells it often shows as a brilliant spot **(Y-fluorescence)**.

R-banding is black where G-bands are dark, and vice versa. Reverse banding is useful if a deletion is suspected in a terminal region which stains pale with G-banding. R-banding is done by thermal denaturation of chromosomes or by BUdR labelling of late-replicating bands.

Silver staining. Silver nitrate stains active nucleolar organizer regions, helping identify chromosomes 13, 14, 15, 21 and 22 in translocations.

G-11 staining. At pH11 Giemsa stains the human and mouse chromosomes differentially in somatic cell hybrids.

The International System for Human Cytogenetic Nomenclature of 1981 **(ISCN 1981)** identifies each chromosome band and sub-band in 400, 550 and 850 band preparations. The chromosome number is followed by p (short arm) or q (long arm) and band numbers, e.g. 1q32.3. 11pter means the tip of the short arm of chromosome 11; Xcen the centromeric region of the X. (*See* p.53 for the location of the main bands on each normal chromosome, and p.66 for the nomenclature of abnormal chromosomes.)

Secondary constrictions are pale-staining apparently uncoiled regions seen on both chromatids of some copies of chromosomes 1, 9 and 16.

Fragile sites resemble secondary constrictions but are seen only when cells are grown in particular conditions. Rare (abnormal) fragile sites are described in chapter 4. About 50

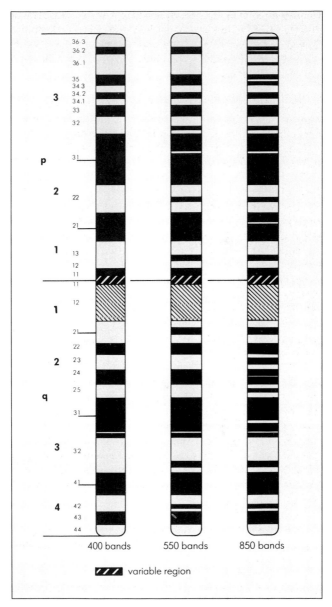

Fig. 2.19 Chromosome 1 showing system for naming bands.

common fragile sites have been described which are present on most or all chromosomes. They become visible after treatment with aphidicolin, and may be hotspots for chromosomal breakage and rearrangement.

LYONIZATION (X-INACTIVATION)

All X chromosomes except one in every cell are permanently condensed and genetically inactive, except for the region of X–Y homology at the tip of the short arm. Lyonization enables cells to function with either one or two X chromosomes without suffering dosage effects (*see* Chapter 4). Inactivation takes place in the embryo at late blastocyst stage. In each XX cell one X, picked at random, is inactivated and the same X is inactive in all the daughters of that cell. The mechanism is believed to be DNA methylation (*see* Chapter 1). In germ-line cells the inactive X is reactivated before meiosis. In mitosis the two X's look similar, but the inactive X replicates later. Females

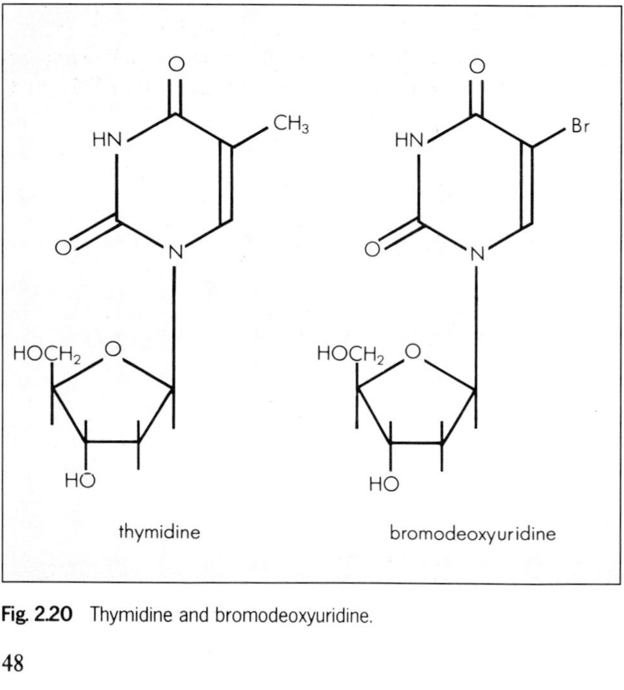

Fig. 2.20 Thymidine and bromodeoxyuridine.

heterozygous for an X-linked character are mosaics of cells expressing the two alleles. This has important consequences in some X-linked diseases (*see* Chapter 5).

The **Barr body** or **sex chromatin** is the inactivated X seen as a dark dot in uncultured (non-dividing) cells. XY and XO cells have no Barr body, XX and XXY have one, XXX have two. This gives a quick but not very reliable sex text which can be done on buccal smears.

Drumsticks in polymorphonuclear cells are projections from the nuclei which correspond to Barr bodies and can be used diagnostically in the same way.

Late replication. All chromosomes replicate during the S phase of the cell cycle, but replication is not entirely synchronous. The inactive X replicates later than the active X, and on autosomes the dark-staining G-bands replicate before pale-staining regions.

Bromodeoxyuridine or **BUdR** is a thymidine analogue which is incorporated into DNA. Late-replicating regions can be pulse-labelled with BUdR late in S phase. Regions so labelled appear dark when stained with a fluorescent dye (Hoechst 33258) and exposed to UV light.

3 Genes, Markers and the Human Genetic Map

Genes may be recognized either as mendelian characters (e.g. the gene for Huntington's disease, whose existence is deduced solely from the mendelian pattern of inheritance), or as DNA sequences coding for some product (e.g. the genes for some collagens have been discovered by molecular biological methods without any disease or abnormality to point the way). Sometimes genes are discovered by cloning and the nature of the product deduced from the DNA sequence. Markers (*see* below) may or may not be genes.

Nomenclature of genes. The names are listed in the proceedings of the biennial Human Gene Mapping Workshops (known as HGM9, and so on and published as special numbers of the journal *Cytogenetics and Cell Genetics*). The naming convention for alleles is often ignored in favour of traditional systems, e.g. HLA-A3. Diseases are often referred to by their number in McKusick's *Mendelian Inheritance in Man* (*see* Chapter 5). DNA probes have local laboratory names, e.g. probe 99-6 defines the locus DXS41.

gene locus symbol		
	APKD	adult onset polycystic kidney disease
	AMY1	amylase (locus 1)
	AMY2	amylase (locus 2)
anonymous DNA segments		
	D10S5	5th one in chromosome 10 catalogue
	DXS164	no.164 on the X
	DXYS1	1st in list of segments present on both X and Y
	DXZ3	3rd in list of repetitive sequences on X
alleles at a locus		
	PGK1*2	2nd allele at PGK1 locus

Fig. 3.1 Nomenclature of loci and alleles.

Alleles are alternative forms of a gene or marker which segregate at meiosis. A person with blood group AB must pass either A or B to each child, but never both. This shows that the A and B genes are allelic.

Locus: this is the site of a gene or marker on a chromosome. The ABO locus on chromosome 9 may carry the A, B or O allele. The concept of a locus, as distinct from the allele which occupies it, is important in mapping and linkage analysis.

Homozygotes have both alleles the same e.g. AA or aa.

Heterozygotes have different alleles e.g. Aa or A_1A_2. Everybody is homozygous at some loci and heterozygous at others.

Hemizygotes have only one allele, e.g. males are hemizygous for loci on the X chromosome.

The genotype is somebody's genetic constitution e.g. AA, Aa.

The phenotype is somebody's observable character, e.g. normal, affected, high-responder.

Dominant characters are expressed in the heterozygote.

Recessive characters are expressed only in the homozygote. Dominance and recessiveness are properties of phenotypes, not of genes: the dominant sickling trait and recessive sickle cell disease are both caused by the same gene. The distinction between dominant and recessive is less clear-cut in X-linked than autosomal conditions, because males are hemizygous, so the question of dominance does not arise, while in females lyonization (*see* Chapter 2) can make the expression in heterozygotes variable.

Codominant characters are both expressed in the heterozygote.

Pleiotropic mutations have many effects. The pleiotropic Bloom's syndrome mutation produces dwarfing, immunodeficiency and chromosomal instability. Most developmental mutations are pleiotropic.

Epistasis means one locus controls the expression of another. ABO is epistatic to secretor, because only people who are not group O can express the secretor phenotype. The opposite to epistasis is **hypostasis**.

Null alleles or **amorphs** are alleles producing no detectable protein. This terminology is used especially in blood grouping, e.g. the Fy and Jk null alleles.

THE HUMAN GENE MAP

The human gene map is produced by a combination of physical and genetic methods. The ultimate aim is a complete nucleotide sequence of the human genome with every gene and marker described. The immediate aims are to have sufficient mapped markers on every chromosome so that linkage analysis can locate any gene, and to locate all mendelian characters relative to these markers. Progress towards these goals has been rapid. About 1,000 structural genes and at least 1,000 anonymous DNA segments have already been mapped.

Genetic maps assign loci to linkage groups and give distances in recombination units (centimorgans). Genetic and physical maps have identical sequences, and each linkage group corresponds to one chromosome, but there is no fixed relation between genetic and physical distance. On average 1cM corresponds to 1Mb in males (less in females), but there are hot-spots and cold-spots for recombination, and regions with more male than female recombination.

Method	Range of resolution
DNA sequencing	1 bp – 10 kb
restriction mapping	0.1 – 100 kb
long range restriction mapping	0.1 – 10 Mb
linkage analysis	0.5 – 20 Mb
somatic cell panels	20 Mb – 1 chromosome

Fig. 3.2 Methods of genetic mapping.

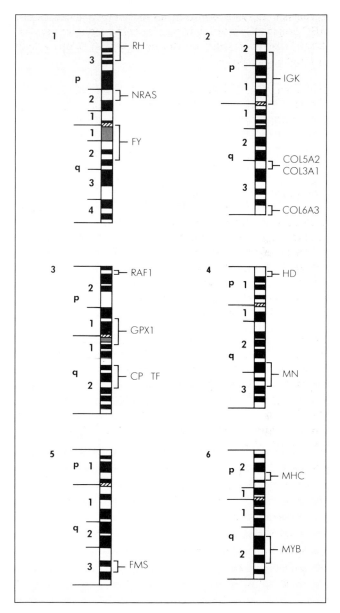

Fig. 3.3 Human genetic map. *(continued over)*

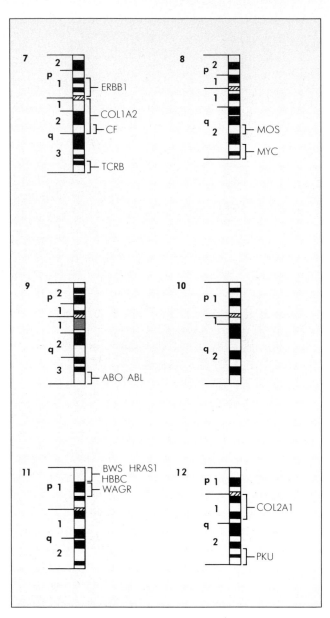

(Only a small selection of mapped loci are shown)

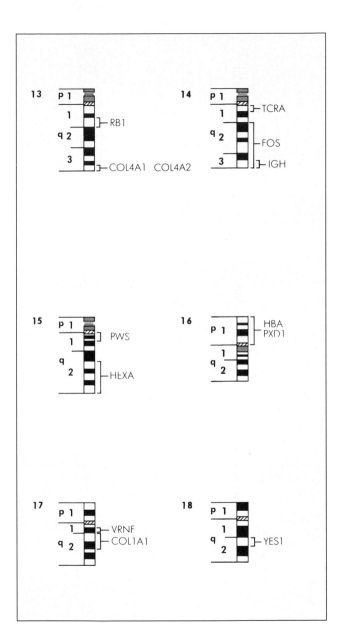

(continued over)

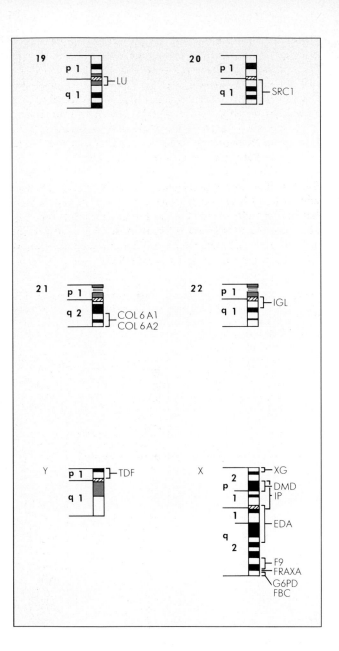

Gene clusters are groups of structurally related genes lying together on a chromosome. They are likely to have arisen by gene duplication. Examples are the HLA and globin clusters and the genes for visual pigments on the X chromosome. Pseudogenes may occur within clustered gene families (e.g. there is a β-globin pseudogene within the β-globin gene cluster), or in unrelated chromosome locations (e.g. the functional dihydrofolate reductase gene is on chromosome 5 and pseudogenes are on chromosomes 3, 6 and 18).

Gene families are groups of genes showing sequence homology and presumably derived from a common ancestor. Most families are dispersed across many chromosomes but some like HLA and the globins are clustered. As nucleotide and amino acid sequence data accumulate it is becoming possible to link most genes into families and superfamilies.

Gene	Symbol	Location
immunoglobin superfamily:		
immunoglobin family:		
Ig heavy chain genes	IGH	14q32.3
kappa light chains	IGK	2p12
lambda light chains	IGL	22q11
T-cell receptor alpha chain	TCRA	14q11
T-cell receptor beta chain	TCRB	7q32
HLA family:		
class I alpha chains	(at least 18 genes)	6p21.3
class II alpha chains	(at least 6 genes)	6p21.3
class II beta chains	(at least 10 genes)	6p21.3
collagen family:		
type I alpha-1 chain	COL1A1	17q21.31
type I alpha-2	COL1A2	7q21.3
type II alpha-1	COL2A1	12q13.1
type III alpha-1	COL3A1	2q31
type IV alpha-1	COL4A1	13q34
type IV alpha-2	COL4A2	13q34
type V alpha-2	COL5A2	2q31
type VI alpha-1	COL6A1	21q223
type VI alpha-2	COL6A2	21q223
type VI alpha-3	COL6A3	2q37

Fig. 3.4 Gene families and superfamilies.

PHYSICAL METHODS OF MAPPING

Physical maps locate genes at cytogenetically defined locations (e.g. 11p15.1) and give distances in bp, kb or Mb. In situ hybridization of probes to chromosome spreads, which is perhaps the most direct method of physical mapping, is described in Chapter 1.

DNA sequencing is the ultimate form of mapping. It is proposed eventually to sequence the entire human genome. DNA fragments up to 1kb long can be sequenced directly. Longer sequences must be assembled from the sequences of a series of overlapping fragments.

Restriction mapping means cutting a piece of DNA (usually a cloned fragment) with a series of restriction enzymes and sizing the fragments by agarose gel electrophoresis. Double digests (two enzymes at once) and partial digests (not every site cut) are used to help relate the fragments. When all the fragments have been successfully arranged in order the result is a restriction map showing the relative positions of recognition sites for each enzyme. Restriction maps are the basic tool for characterizing DNA at the kilobase level. If part of the same restriction map is found in two independent clones, the two probably overlap. The map in Fig. 3.5 (of sequences near the complement C4 genes) suggests this sequence is a diverged tandem repeat: the map from 30–60kb closely resembles the map from 0–30kb but is not identical to it.

Long range restriction mapping means using rare-cutter enzymes to generate very large fragments which can be separated and sized by pulsed field electrophoresis. These methods enable sequences of several megabases to be restriction mapped, and close the gap between the size ranges of restriction mapping and chromosomal techniques such as in situ hybridization and deletion mapping.

Chromosome walking means isolating genomic sequences adjacent to a given clone by screening a library for clones whose restriction maps overlap. A multi-step walk might eventually cover several hundred kilobases.

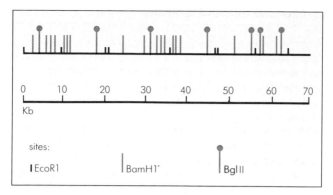

Fig. 3.5 Restriction map.

Chromosome jumping is accelerated chromosome walking, using specialized cloning techniques to move hundreds of kilobases at a time. The technique is novel and rather speculative.

Deletion mapping means studying people with chromosomal deletions to find deleted genes or markers. On autosomes deletions unmask recessive characters: a Pp heterozygote will show the p phenotype if P is deleted. Thus if the same recessive disease is seen in two unrelated people who happen both to have a deletion of the same chromosomal region, the disease gene probably maps to this region. The frequent association of retinoblastoma with deletion of 13q14 pointed to the location of the retinoblastoma gene. On the X chromosome, males with deletions have the diseases whose genes map in the deleted segment, and their DNA does not hybridize with probes located in that segment. In hybrid cell lines a series of overlapping deletions can be used to order a set of probes on a chromosome.

Hybrid cell panels are collections of mouse cell lines each containing a known small selection of human chromosomes. They are the main tool for mapping genes to particular chromosomes or chromosomal regions. Lines which produce a human gene product, or whose DNA hybridizes with a human-specific probe, are identified and their human chromosome content compared.

The cell lines are made by growing human and mouse cells together in the presence of agents which destabilize cell membranes. This induces them to fuse. The resulting hetero-karyons are unstable and tend selectively to shed human chromosomes. Eventually stable cell lines result which contain the full mouse genome but only a few human chromosomes. These can be characterized cytogenetically by G-11 banding. Hybrids for mapping to sub-chromosomal regions are made from human cells with translocations or deletions.

human chromosomes \ hybrid cell line	1	2	3	4	5	6	7	8	9	10	11	12	human control	mouse control
1							+	+					+	
2	+	+	+	+	+								+	
3	+	+	+	+	+		+	+	+				+	
4							+	+	+				+	
5													+	
6	+	+	+	+									+	
7													+	
8	+	+											+	
9													+	
10	+	+	+	+	+		+						+	
11	+			+	+	+					+		+	
12	+	+	+	+	+	+	+						+	
13				+	+								+	
14	+			+	+		+						+	
15	+												+	
16	+												+	
17	+												+	
18				+		+							+	
19	+			+	+	+							+	
20	+	+	+	+	+	+							+	
21	+			+	+				+				+	
22	+	+							+				+	
X	+	+	+	+	+	+	+	+	+		+		+	
	✓	✓	✓	✓	✓	✓	✓	✗	✗	✗	✗	✗	✓	✗
hybridization of cloned DNA														

Fig. 3.6 Mapping using a hybrid cell panel.

LINKAGE ANALYSIS

Linkage analysis uses pedigree data to discover whether loci are linked and to estimate the recombination fraction.

Linked markers segregate together in meiosis more often than expected by chance, because they lie close together on the same chromosome.

Syntenic means on the same chromosome. Syntenic markers may not show linkage, if they lie far apart. Synteny is established by studies of hybrid cell panels.

Recombination fraction is the proportion of recombinants. For unlinked loci it is 0.5, for linked loci between 0 and 0.5.

Mapping functions relate the genetic distance between two loci to the observed recombination fraction. However great the distance, the recombination fraction will not exceed 0.5 because of multiple crossovers. The simplest mapping function is Haldane's function:

$$w = 1/2\,(1-2\ln(r))\text{ or }r = 1/2\,(1-e^{-2w})$$

(w = distance in Morgans, r = recombination fraction).

Interference is the tendency of a crossover to affect the probability of a second crossover nearby. Positive interference means that one crossover inhibits the formation of others near it. Negative interference means that very close multiple crossovers may be favoured, but this is not known to occur in man.

Exclusion mapping means using negative linkage data to work out where a locus is *not*. With sufficient negative linkage data a locus can be excluded from whole chromosomes or even from most of the genome. This enables the search to be concentrated on the remaining non-excluded locations.

Recombinants are children who inherit a different combination of alleles at two loci from the gametes which made the parents. In Fig. 3.7 II$_1$ was formed by a sperm carrying A1,B1 and an egg carrying A2,B2. His children who inherit A1,B1 or A2,B2 from him are non-recombinants, but those who inherit A1,B2 or A2,B1 are recombinants. Recombination between linked loci is the result of chromosomal crossing over in meiosis.

Phase or **linkage phase** is the relation (coupling or repulsion) between alleles at two linked loci. Alleles on the same physical chromosome (such as A1 and B1 in individual II$_1$ of Fig. 3.7) are in **coupling**; alleles on opposite chromosomes (such as A1 and B2 in this person) are in **repulsion**.

Phase-known double heterozygotes are those where we know which alleles are in coupling and which in repulsion. This is determined from studying other family members. Linkage analysis is more efficient with phase-known parents because recombinant children can be identified unambiguously.

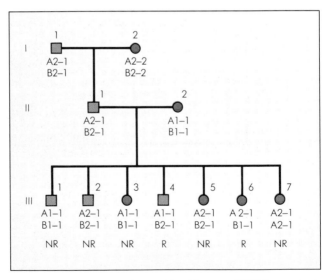

Fig. 3.7 Pedigree with recombinants. (A and B are two RLFP's.)

Lod scores are the statistical outcome of linkage analysis in man. They are the logarithm (base 10) of an odds ratio:

$$\text{odds} \quad \frac{\text{the two loci are linked with recombination fraction } \theta}{\text{the two loci are unlinked (recombination fraction 0.5)}}$$

Human linkage analysis requires elaborate methods because families are small and pedigree structures rarely ideal. Lod scores are calculated by computer programs from the pedigree data. The end result is a table or graph of lods at various recombination fractions. A lod score of +3.0 or greater is statistically significant evidence of linkage. The curve in Fig. 3.8 shows a peak lod score of 4.3 at $\theta = 0.05$; the confidence intervals are the recombination fractions at which the lod is one unit below the peak (0.025 and 0.10). A lod score less than −2.0 is evidence against linkage. Lod scores between −2 and +3 are inconclusive. The lower curve in Fig. 3.8 excludes linkage closer than $\theta = 0.10$ but is inconclusive for greater recombination fractions. A great advantage of lod scores is that they can be summed across families.

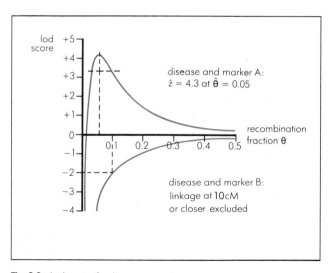

Fig. 3.8 Lod scores for disease vs marker.

z and θ are the lod score and recombination fraction; **ẑ** and **θ̂** are the values of z and θ at the peak in the lod score curve.

Multilocus mapping. Multi-point crosses are much more efficient than two-point crosses for deciding the order of a set of linked loci. Double recombinants can often be identified directly, whereas in two-point analysis they appear to be non-recombinant. A series of multipoint analyses has been used in man to establish a framework of ordered RRLPs for each chromosome, which can then be used in families with interesting diseases to map the disease locus.

Location scores are the equivalent in multilocus mapping of lod scores in two-point mapping. They are twice the natural logarithm of the likelihood ratio:

unknown locus at this location within the marker framework
unknown locus right outside marker framework

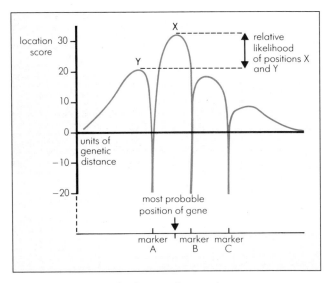

Fig. 3.9 Location scores for disease vs three markers.

Sib-pair analysis is a simple form of linkage analysis used for mapping (usually exclusion mapping) of autosomal recessive diseases and for searching for susceptibility genes for diseases with non-mendelian inheritance (*see* Chapter 7). The starting material is a collection of 20–100 pairs of sibs both of whom suffer from the disease under study.

For any locus the probabilities that two sibs share 0, 1 or 2 of the parental alleles are 1/4, 1/2 and 1/4 respectively. If pairs of affected sibs show a persistent tendency to share one particular chromosomal segment more often than this random expectation, the probable reason is that the segment carries a gene conferring susceptibility to the disease.

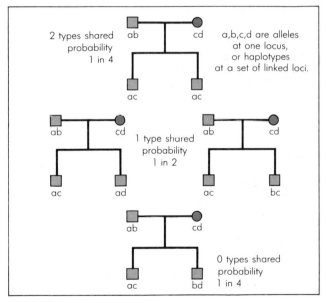

Fig. 3.10 Expected sharing of alleles by pairs of sibs.

4 | Chromosome Abnormalities

Nomenclature of abnormalities describes the appearance under the microscope, not necessarily the events at the DNA level. Apparent breakpoints are described as simple cut-and-join events, although at the DNA level there might be small deletions, duplications or inversions of flanking material. Since the only landmarks on chromosomes are the boundaries of dark and light bands, breakpoints can never be localized more accurately than to a single pair of dark and light bands. For example if a deletion removes one dark band and some neighbouring light-staining material from the middle of a chromosome arm, it is impossible to say how much of the missing light-stained material comes from above or below the dark band.

The nomenclature of any given abnormality should state:
- the number of chromosomes
- the sex chromosome constitution (e.g. XX, XY)
- the type of abnormality (e.g. translocation, deletion; optionally the type of translocation can be specified as rcp or rob)
- the chromosome bands and sub-bands involved.

A more complex nomenclature of structural abnormalities exists with double (::) or single colons used to specify breakage with and without rejoining.

Constitutional abnormalities are present throughout the body. They result from an abnormal gamete, abnormal fertilization or an abnormal event in the early embryo.

Somatic or acquired abnormalities are present only in a few cells or tissues. The zygote was normal, and the abnormality was acquired at some later stage. Somatic abnormalities include many which would be lethal if constitutional.

Abnormality	Example of nomenclature
Numerical:	
euploid	
triploidy	69,XXY
aneuploid	
monosomy	45,X
trisomy	47,XY,+21
mixoploid	45,X/46,XX
Structural:	
deletion	
terminal	46,XY,del(18)(q21→qter)
interstitial	46,XX,del(12)(p13.1→p13.3)
duplication	46,XX,dup(14)(q31→qter)
ring chromosome	46,XY,r(20)(p13q13)
isochromosome	46,X,i(Xq)
translocation	
reciprocal	46,XX,t(4;12)(p16;p13.3)
Robertsonian	45,XY,−13,−14,+t(13q;14q)
inversion	
pericentric	46,XY,inv(1)(p31q43)
paracentric	46,XX,inv(1)(q23q42)
fragile site	46,XY,fra(Xq27)
polymorphic variant	
extra heterochromatin	1qh+
large satellite	15ps+
Unidentified or unspecified material:	
additional chromosome	47,XY + marker
chromosome arm too big	18p+
chromosome arm too small	18p−

Fig. 4.1 Classification and nomenclature of chromosome abnormalities.

Numerical abnormalities occur when a wrong number of copies of one or more chromosomes is present. Few are compatible with survival if every cell is affected.

Euploid means having one or more complete set of chromosomes. The set is symbolized by n. Euploid cells have e.g. n, 2n, 3n chromosomes. For humans n = 23.

Aneuploid means not euploid. Constitutionally aneuploid humans have 45 or 47 chromosomes, rarely 48 or 49, but cancer cells often show extreme and bizarre aneuploidy. Aneuploidy arises from non-disjunction of chromosomes during cell division.

Triploidy occurs in perhaps 2% of human conceptuses but almost all die *in utero* and the few which survive to term do not live long. Triploids arise from a failure of meiosis or abnormal fertilization. Triploidy is lethal probably because of gene dosage imbalance between the X-chromosome and autosomes.

Condition	Karyotype	Syndrome name	Frequency at birth
Compatible with long term survival:			
Trisomy 21	47,XX or XY,+21	Down Syndrome	1/ 600
Trisomy X	47,XXX	Triple-X	1/1,000♀
XXY	47,XXY	Klinefelter	1/ 800♂
XYY	47,XYY	XYY syndrome	1/1,000♂
Monosomy X	45,X	Turner	1/10,000♀
Leading to stillbirth or neonatal death:			
Triploidy	69,XXX, XXY or XYY		v.rare
Trisomy 13	47,XX or XY,+13	Patau's	1/5,000
Trisomy 18	47,XX or XY,+18	Edwards	1/3,000

Fig. 4.2 Numerical abnormalities seen in full-term infants.

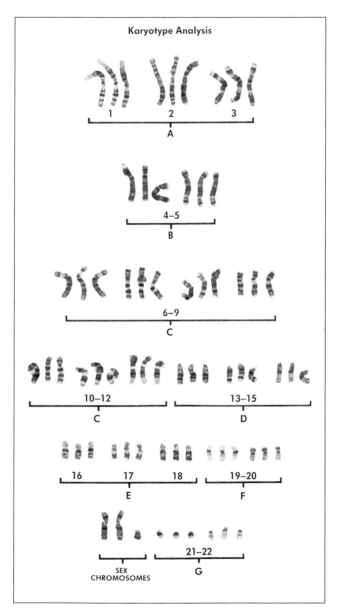

Fig. 4.3 Triploid karyotype.

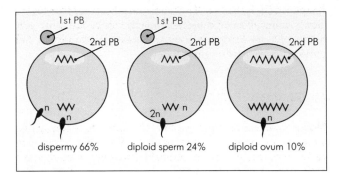

Fig. 4.4 Origins of triploidy.

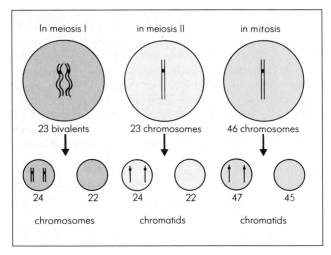

Fig. 4.5 Non-disjunction (the chromosomes which disjoin normally are not shown).

Non-disjunction means a failure of chromosomes or chromatids to disjoin as they should at anaphase. In the first or second meiotic division this results in gametes with one chromosome too few or too many, which produce monosomic or trisomic zygotes. Thus trisomy 13 and 21 arise by non-disjunction in paternal meiosis I (12% of cases) and II (5%) or maternal meiosis I (68%) and II (15%). Mitotic non-disjunction produces mosaics.

Anaphase lag is the loss of a chromosome because it moves too slowly at anaphase of cell division, and fails to reach the pole before the nuclear membrane reforms. Chromosomes left outside the nucleus are broken down.

AUTOSOMAL ANEUPLOIDY

Monosomic cells have a single copy of one chromosome (giving a total of 45 chromosomes in man). Monosomy is common in early embryos, but no autosomal monosomy is compatible with survival except as a mosaic.

Trisomic cells have three copies of one chromosome (giving a total of 47 chromosomes in man). There are 22 possible autosomal trisomies in man (trisomy 1, trisomy 2, and so on). All 22 have been seen in eggs fertilized *in vitro* or early embryos. All except trisomies 1 and 19 have been detected in spontaneous abortions. Apparent constitutional trisomies 7, 8, 14, 16 and 22 have been reported in 8–12 week pregnancies sampled by chorion villus biopsy. In non-mosaic liveborn infants only trisomies 13, 18 and 21 are commonly seen. Trisomies 7, 8, 9, 10, 15, 16, 20 and 22 have been reported in individual liveborn infants but there must be some doubt about these diagnoses.

Double trisomy means simultaneous trisomy for two chromosomes, e.g. 48, XX, +18, +21. Double trisomy may be the coincidental result of two independent accidents, but may reflect a more generalized disturbance of meiosis.

Partial trisomy means trisomy for part of a chromosome. The usual cause is unbalanced segregation in a balanced translocation carrier. Do not confuse partial trisomy (every cell is trisomic for part of the chromosome) with mosaic trisomy (some cells normal, some trisomic for the whole chromosome).

Tetrasomy means four copies of one chromosome. Complete autosomal tetrasomy is not seen. Partial tetrasomy may occur if there is an extra isochromosome, e.g. the dicentric i(22pter →q11) in cat-eye syndrome.

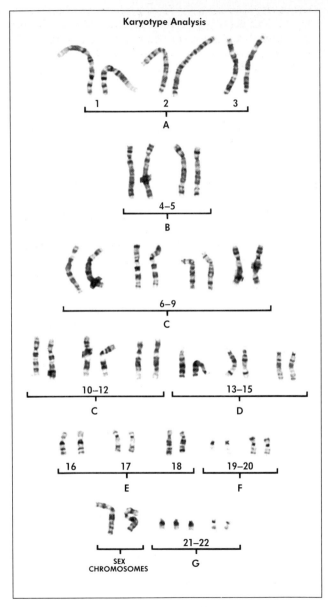

Fig. 4.6 Karyotype of an autosomal trisomy (21).

Dosage effects are changes of phenotype due to changes in the number of copies of a gene. Chromosome 21 carries the gene for superoxide dismutase, and trisomy 21 cells produce 50% more of this enzyme than normal cells. Dosage effects in regulatory products can produce qualitative changes in phenotype.

Chromosomal imbalance refers to the pathological effect of extra or missing chromosomes, which is presumably due to multiple dosage effects.

SEX CHROMOSOME ABNORMALITIES

Sex chromosome aneuploidy is tolerated much better than autosomal aneuploidy because special mechanisms minimise dosage effects. These have evolved to allow normal development regardless whether a person is XX or XY. The Y chromosome carries little except male-determining genes, and extra

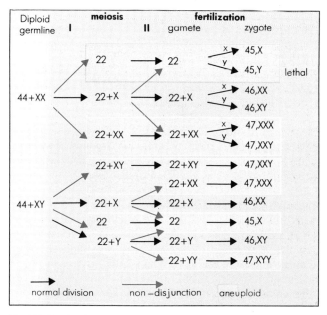

Fig. 4.7 Results of non-disjunction of sex chromosomes.

copies have minimal effect. For the X chromosome, lyonization ensures that there is only one active X per cell, regardless
of the number in the karyotype. This dosage compensation
does not occur in the very early embryo, in meiotic cells or for
the tip of Xp, hence X chromosome aneuploidy is not without
some phenotypic effects.

XY females occur when the male-determining process fails. All
mammals develop as females unless positively switched to
maleness. The commonest cause of XY females is **testicular
feminisation syndrome** due to an X-linked defect of androgen
receptors.

XX males occur with a frequency of 1 in 20,000. Most have the
testis-determining gene TDF transferred from its normal position on Yp to Xp, demonstrable by hybridization to Y-specific
DNA probes. This transfer occurs when the normal crossover
in the homologous region of the X and Y takes place at an
abnormally proximal location. Rarely, no Y material is
demonstrable.

Hermaphrodites have both testicular and ovarian tissue.
Karyotypes reported include 46,XX, 46,XX/46,XY and 46,XY.

Mixoploidy describes the coexistence of two or more chromosomally different cell lines without specifying whether they
represent mosaicism or chimaerism.

Mosaics have two or more genetically different cell lines derived from a single zygote. Chromosomal mosaics arise in one
of the mitotic divisions of the early embryo by non-disjunction
or by chromosome loss through anaphase lag.

Diploid/triploid mosaics are a special case because mitotic
non-disjunction is a very unlikely mechanism for gaining or
losing a balanced set of 23 chromosomes. Most probably they
result from fusion of the second polar body with one of the
cleavage nuclei of a normal diploid zygote.

Chimaeras contain two or more cell lines originating from
different zygotes. **Dispermic chimaeras** result from complete
fusion of dizygotic twins. **Blood chimaeras** arise when ana-

stomoses of placental vessels allow cells from one twin to colonise a co-twin. XX/XY chimaeras may be intersexes; otherwise they are often phenotypically normal and escape detection unless blood grouping reveals, for instance, a mixture of A and B cells.

Risk of trisomy in the baby of a chromosomally normal couple depends mainly on maternal age. It is controversial whether there is any paternal age effect, but it is certainly small compared to the maternal effect. Probably this is related to the chance of bivalents falling apart during the long prophase in female meiosis. Proper segregation requires intact bivalents.

Recurrence risk of trisomies, though low, is greater than the risk with no family history, e.g. about 1% for Down's syndrome at age 25 when both parents are chromosomally normal. This may be because of undetected mosaicism, or because there is a genetically determined tendency to non-disjunction. Translocation carriers may have a substantially higher risk, see below.

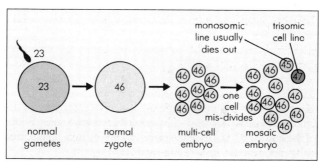

Fig. 4.8 Origin of mosaic trisomy cell lines.

Chromosomally normal couple, no history of Down's Syndrome					
Age of mother	25	30	35	40	42
Risk of Down's	1/2000	1/1000	1/500	1/100	1/50

Fig. 4.9 Risk of a Down's syndrome child.

Risk of Turner's syndrome unlike trisomies is unrelated to maternal age, and the recurrence risk is probably no higher than the population risk.

Hydatidiform moles are abnormal conceptuses in which the membranes but no fetus develops. There are two types, complete and partial. **Complete moles** have two paternal and no maternal genomes. **Partial moles** are often triploid, with two paternal and one maternal genomes. They are believed to be accidents of fertilization and not related to any parental genetic or chromosomal condition.

Dermatoglyphics is the study of fingerprints, palm prints and such like. Chromosomal abnormalities disturb the normal pattern. In the past these changes were intensively studied, but little clinical use is now made of dermatoglyphics.

STRUCTURAL ABNORMALITIES

Structural abnormalities include deletions, duplications, inversions and translocations. Examples are shown below, with their probable origin through faulty repair of chromosome breaks. Alternative mechanisms are aberrant recombination, or by chromosome replication hopping from one template to another.

Balanced structural abnormalities have no extra or missing material overall. As long as the correct material is present in the cell, the way it is packaged into chromosomes is important only in meiosis. Thus balanced abnormalities rarely have any phenotypic effect on the patient. The chromosomes behave normally in mitosis, but in meiosis unbalanced gametes may be produced. Balanced chromosomal abnormalities are a significant cause of infertility, recurrent abortions or abnormal babies in phenotypically normal people.

X-autosome translocations are an exception to the rule that balanced abnormalities have no phenotypic effects. In female carriers the structurally normal X is preferentially inactivated, because in cells which inactivate the translocated X the inactivation spreads into the autosomal material, causing effective monosomy and cell death. If the translocation breakpoint disrupts a gene, the carrier will manifest the corresponding disease. The location of the breakpoint thus points to the location of the gene for the disease. The Duchenne muscular dystrophy gene at Xp21 is particularly vulnerable because it is so large (2Mb).

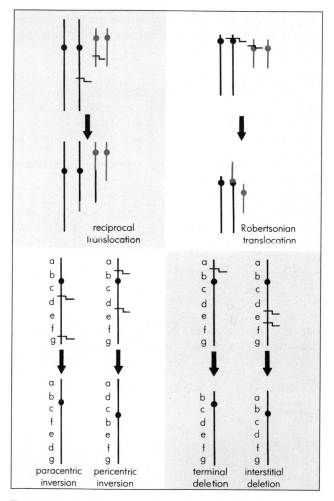

Fig. 4.10 Structural chromosome abnormalities and their origin.

Reciprocal translocations happen when two chromosomes exchange non-homologous segments. Carriers are usually phenotypically normal, but they are at risk of having abnormal children. At pachytene of meiosis the translocated chromosomes and their non-translocated homologues pair up in a cross-shaped figure, with matching sequences synapsed. Several different segregation patterns are possible at anaphase, some of which produce chromosomally abnormal gametes. Unbalanced segregation in a translocation carrier produces a conceptus with both partial monosomy and partial trisomy.

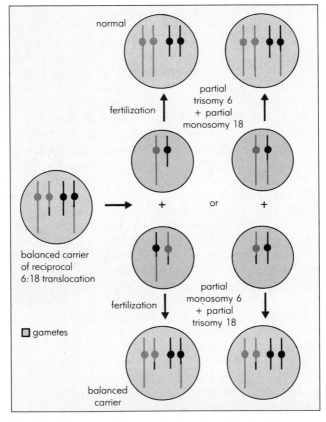

Fig. 4.11 Meiotic products in a carrier of a reciprocal translocation.

Robertsonian translocations happen when two of the acrocentric chromosomes (usually numbers 13 or 14, less often numbers 15, 21 or 22) fuse at or near the centromere. The short arms are lost, but this does not produce any phenotypic effect, hence these are regarded as balanced abnormalities. The translocated chromosome is often dicentric, but segregates regularly at cell division, probably because the two centromeres are so close together. As with balanced reciprocal translocations, carriers are at risk of conceiving chromosomally abnormal offspring. In this case the abnormality is a complete trisomy or complete monosomy.

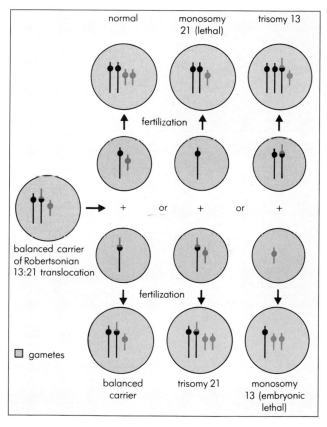

Fig. 4.12 Meiotic products in a carrier of a Robertsonian translocation.

Translocation Down's syndrome is due to segregation of a Robertsonian translocation, usually t(14:21). Clinically it is indistinguishable from trisomic Down's, but the recurrence risk is much higher if one of the parents carries the translocation. About 4% of Down's are this type.

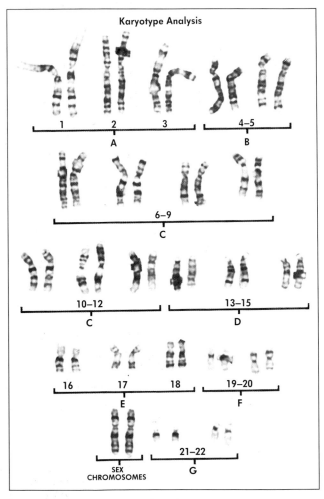

Fig. 4.13 Karyotype of a balanced translocation carrier 46,XX,t(4:11)(q31;p13).

Insertional translocations insert a block of material from one chromosome into an interstitial site on another. Children of carriers are at risk of partial monosomy (**interstitial deletion**) or partial trisomy.

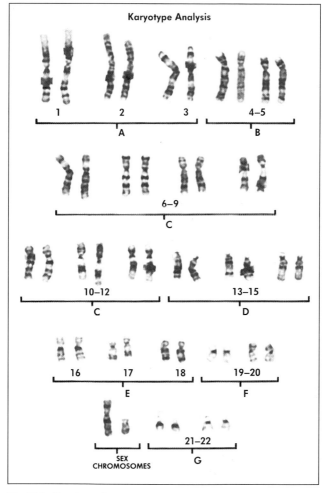

Fig. 4.14 Karyotype of unbalanced translocation 46,XY,der(11), son of balanced carrier in Fig. 4.13.

Paracentric inversions do not include the centromere in the inverted segment. Chromosomal morphology is unaffected, but the inversion may be revealed by an abnormal banding pattern. They are balanced abnormalities with no phenotypic effect except sometimes reduced fertility (crossovers produce grossly unbalanced gametes which do not survive).

Pericentric inversions include the centromere in the inverted segment. The inversion usually alters the chromosome morphology.

Inversion loops are structures seen at pachytene when a chromosome carrying an inversion synapses with a structurally normal homologue. They form only with large inversions, and not always then; the alternative is a linear partially mismatched structure. If a crossover occurs within an inversion loop, the recombinant chromosomes are abnormal. Crossing over in a paracentric inversion loop produces dicentric and acentric recombinant chromosomes, which are likely to be lost by anaphase lag. Crossing over in a pericentric inversion loop produces chromosomes with terminal duplications and deficiencies, which may result in abnormal offspring.

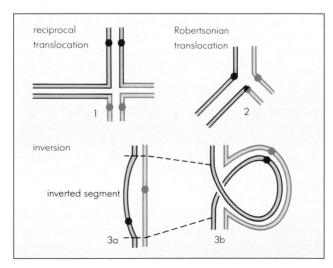

Fig. 4.15 Meiotic pairing.

Deletions can be interstitial or terminal, although the necessity for a functional telomere may mean that only ring chromosomes have truly terminal deletions.

Microdeletions are deletions at or below the limit of microscopic resolution. Even the smallest visible deletions remove many megabases of DNA and usually produce the multi system syndromes characteristic of chromosomal anomalies. DNA technology is revealing many submicroscopic deletions.

Ring chromosomes are a special class of deleted chromosome, easily recognizable cytogenetically, which have lost both ends and joined up in a circle. A ring chromosome will be unstable if the daughter rings are interlocked after replication.

Duplications can be tandem or inverted, and like deletions they range in size from molecular to cytogenetic. Large duplications behave as partial trisomies. Duplications of one or a few complete genes may cause dosage effects. Duplication of a small portion of a gene is likely to destroy its function by generating a frame-shift or disrupting RNA splicing.

Isochromosomes are abnormal metacentric (rarely dicentric) chromosomes consisting of duplicated long arms or duplicated short arms of one chromosome. A woman with 46,X,i(Xq) is trisomic for the long arm and monosomic for the short arm of the X. They are supposed to arise by misdivision of the centromere so that one daughter cell gets both long arms and the other gets both short arms.

Double minutes are small extra chromosomes typically seen in highly evolved cells which have been subject to strong selection, such as cancer cells or drug-resistant cell lines. They carry many copies of one gene. For example methotrexate resistant cells contain amplified dihydrofolate reductase genes often in the form of double minutes.

Homogeneously staining regions are similar to double minutes, but inserted into a normal chromosome.

Marker chromosomes are unidentified or unspecified abnormal chromosomes, e.g. a cell with an extra chromosome whose origin has not been identified might be described as 47,XY,+marker.

Chromosome deletion syndromes are rarely well defined because of the infinite variety of partial monosomies which is possible. Some clinically well defined syndromes, such as Prader–Willi syndrome, are often but not always associated with a particular microdeletion. It is assumed that patients with no visible chromosomal abnormality have either a submicroscopic deletion or else a point mutation at the same position.

Chromosome duplication syndromes are uncommon. Partial trisomy due to unbalanced segregation in a translocation carrier and partial tetrasomy due to an isochromosome, are commoner than chromosomal duplications.

Syndrome	Chromosomal abnormality
Wolf–Hirschhorn	variable size deletion of 4p16
cri du chat	variable deletion of 5p14-5pter
Prader–Willi	often deletion of 15q11-q13
Angelman	often deletion of 15q11-q13
retinoblastoma	sometimes deletion of 13q14
Wilms tumour–aniridia	sometimes deletion of 11p13
Beckwith–Wiedemann	often duplication of 11p15
cat-eye	extra iso(22pter→q11)

Fig. 4.16 Syndromes associated with small chromosomal anomalies.

Chromosome heteromorphisms are harmless though visible differences between homologous chromosomes, useful as markers e.g. for determining which parent contributed the extra chromosome to a trisomic child.

Polymorphic variants are common chromosome heteromorphisms. They include:
- extra centromeric heterochromatin in chromosomes 1, 9 or 16 (1qh+, 9qh+, 16qh+).
- presence or absence, and size, of the satellites on the acrocentric chromosomes 13, 14, 15, 21, 22.
- size variation in the heterochromatic long arm of the Y.
- a small pericentric inversion in chromosome 9 (inv(9)).
- variable quinacrine fluorescence at the centromeres of chromosomes 3 and 4.

FRAGILE X SYNDROME

Rare fragile sites are seen as unstained gaps in chromosomes when cells are put under some stress. Unlike the common fragile sites (*see* Chapter 2) they are present in only a few people. About 20 have been described. They are classified into folate-sensitive, distamycin A-inducible and bromodeoxyuridine-inducible sites. With the exception of the folate-sensitive fragile site at Xq27, they have no phenotypic effect.

Fragile-X syndrome is moderate to severe mental retardation in males, often with large testes and a characteristic face, associated with the rare fragile site at Xq27. It is transmitted through families as an X-linked mendelian condition (locus symbol FRAXA). About one third of female carriers show some degree of retardation. 1/1000 males are affected: it is the commonest cause of moderate mental retardation in males, after Down's syndrome.

Both the fragile site and the mental retardation are presumed to be consequences of some unknown molecular event. In some families a clinically identical X-linked syndrome is seen without any fragile X. The fragile X is seen only when cells are cultured in folate-deficient medium, and only in a proportion of cells. The percentage of cells showing the fragile X does not vary greatly in successive tests on the same subject. Some

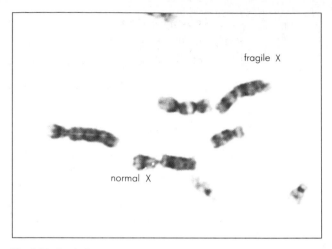

fragile X

normal X

Fig. 4.17 Fragile X.

pedigrees start with a mentally normal male obligate carrier, and it has been surmised that such 'normal transmitting males' may carry some form of premutation, which requires transmission through a female for it to be converted into the pathological form (perhaps by recombination, or as a consequence of lyonization).

CANCER CYTOGENETICS

Over 125 consistently occurring structural chromosome changes have been described associated with specific malignancies, including translocations, deletions and iso-chromosomes. Bizarre abnormal karyotypes are frequently seen in cancer cells, and the tumour-specific changes have to be disentangled from the many non-specific changes.

Tumour-specific breakpoints in translocations and deletions may point to the locations of causative genes. About 125 specific breakpoints have been recognized, involving all chromosomes except the Y. Breaks in specific chromosome regions are associated with at least 20 different types of solid tumours, 15 haematological malignancies and 4 benign tumours.

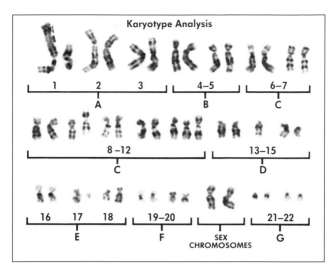

Fig. 4.18 Bizarre karyotype of cancer cell.

Breakpoint	Tumour
1q36	MDS, ANLL, neuroblastoma
1q21	ANLL, carcinoma of bladder, uterus, breast
3p21-p13	carcinoma of lung, kidney and ovary
3q21, 3q26	MDS, ANLL, MPS
	inv(3)(q21q26); t(3:3)(q21;q26) etc
9q34	ANLL, MPS, CML, ALL
	(site of abl oncogene)
11q23	ALL, ANLL, MDS
	(site of ets1 oncogene)
13q14	retinoblastoma, alveolar rhabdomyosarcoma
14q11	malignant T-cell proliferation
	(site of T-cell receptor gene)
14q32	malignant B-cell proliferation
	(site of immunoglobin gene)

MDS = myelodysplastic syndrome
ANLL = acute nonlymphocytic leukaemia
MPS = myeloproliferative syndrome
CML = chronic myeloid leukaemia
ALL = acute lymphatic leukaemia

Fig. 4.19 Examples of tumour-specific breakpoints.

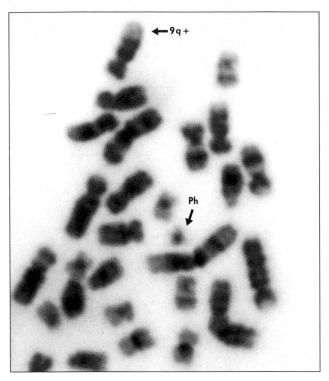

Fig. 4.20 Ph chromosome.

Philadelphia or Ph chromosome is a small marker chromosome which is diagnostic of chronic myeloid leukaemia. It is a derivative of chromosome 22, produced by a reciprocal 9:22 translocation which brings the c-abl oncogene on chromosome 9 into juxtaposition with a gene caller bcr.

CHROMATID ABNORMALITIES

Chromatid abnormalities arise in S or G_2 phase of the cell cycle, when the chromosome consists of two chromatids. They affect single cells; if stable, they will appear after the next S phase as chromosome aberrations.

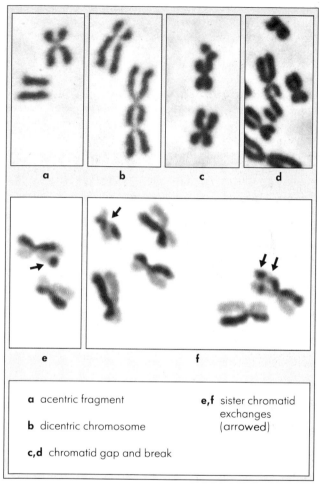

Fig. 4.21 Chromatid abnormalities.

a acentric fragment

b dicentric chromosome

c,d chromatid gap and break

e,f sister chromatid exchanges (arrowed)

Sister chromatid exchanges (SCE's) are reciprocal exchanges between the two chromatids of a chromosome. They are seen in normal cells, but at much increased frequencies in cells which have been exposed to radiation or mutagens. The SCE score is therefore an indicator of chromosome damage. To see SCE's, chromosomes must be harlequin stained (Fig. 4.21e, f).

Harlequin staining is done by exposing synchronized cell cultures to bromodeoxyuridine (BUdR, *see* Chapter 2) for two rounds of DNA replication, and then staining with the fluorescent dye Hoechst 33258 and exposing to UV light. DNA with BUdR in both strands stains lighter.

Non-sister chromatid exchanges are the counterpart at the chromatid level of reciprocal translocations. In mitotic spreads they show cross-shaped figures similar to those shown by translocations at diplotene of meiosis.

Chromatid gaps are small unstained gaps in one chromatid. Gaps (Fig. 4.21c) differ from **chromatid breaks** (Fig. 4.21d) because in gaps the fragment does not fall off at anaphase.

Chromosomal instability syndromes are genetic diseases in which patients show a high frequency of chromosomal abnormalities, different in every cell, as though the cells had been irradiated. The main ones are ataxia telangiectasia, Fanconi's anaemia and Bloom's syndrome.

PEDIGREE PATTERNS

Sibs are brothers or sisters.

Half-sibs have one parent in common.

Cousins or **first cousins** are the children of sibs. The loose usage of cousin to mean relative or kinsman is not allowed in genetics.

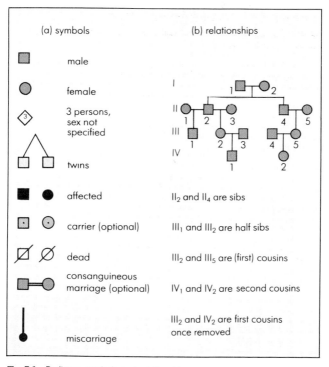

(a) symbols

☐ male

◯ female

◇ 3 persons, sex not specified

△ twins

■ ● affected

☐ ◉ carrier (optional)

☒ ⊘ dead

☐—◯ consanguineous marriage (optional)

| miscarriage

(b) relationships

II₂ and II₄ are sibs

III₁ and III₂ are half sibs

III₂ and III₅ are (first) cousins

IV₁ and IV₂ are second cousins

III₂ and IV₂ are first cousins once removed

Fig. 5.1 Pedigree symbols and relationships.

Second cousins are people whose parents are first cousins.

Consanguineous marriages are marriages between blood relatives. The term has no absolute meaning since all humans are ultimately related; it is used to draw attention to an unusually close relationship. The degree of consanguinity is measured by the coefficient of relationship or kinship (*see* Chapter 8).

Mendelian characters follow one of the pedigree patterns shown opposite. These patterns are caused by the segregation of a single pair of alleles located on an autosome or the X chromosome which govern a dominant, codominant or recessive phenotype. About 4,000 are known, plus at least another 1,000 RFLPs which follow mendelian patterns.

Pseudoautosomal describes the pattern of inheritance of markers located in the pairing region at the tip of the short arms of the X and Y chromosomes. Such markers follow an apparently autosomal pedigree pattern.

A marker is any mendelian character used to follow the transmission of a segment of a chromosome through a pedigree. A good marker must be highly polymorphic (ideally everybody should be heterozygous), codominant (so that genotypes can always be inferred from phenotypes) and easily scored in readily available tissue. The most usual markers are DNA RFLPs (*see* Chapter 1); others include blood groups, protein polymorphisms, tissue types and polymorphic variants of chromosomes (*see* Chapter 2).

Polymorphism information content (PIC) of a marker is a measure of how useful a marker is for tracking a gene in a pedigree. PIC ranges from 0 (useless) to 1 (always fully informative). It is a function of the number of alleles and their frequency. If there are n alleles and the ith allele has frequency p_i, the PIC is

$$1 - \sum_{i=1}^{n} p_i^2 - \sum_{i=1}^{n-1} \sum_{j=i+1}^{n} 2p_i^2 p_j^2$$

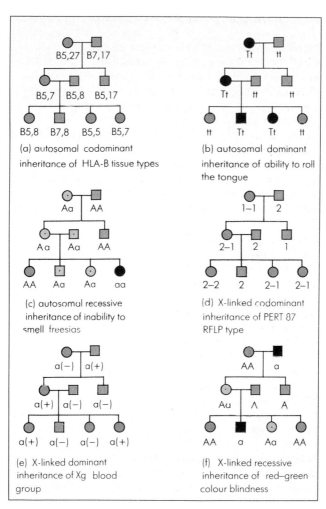

Fig. 5.2 Mendelian patterns.

Autosomal dominant	1541 definite + 1120 probable
Autosomal recessive	628 definite + 864 probable
X-linked	143 definite + 173 probable

Fig. 5.3 Numbers of mendelian phenotypes.

Blood groups refer to antigens on the surface of red cells. **Private groups** are found in one or a few families, **public groups** are polymorphic in the general population. Blood groups were the first major set of mendelian markers to be discovered in man. A vast body of information is available on the distribution of blood groups in every human population. Most systems have additional rare antigens not listed in Fig. 5.4. Antigens discovered as rare variants in Caucasians sometimes turn out to be much more frequent in other populations.

Protein polymorphisms or **electromorphs** are usually observed as differences in electrophoretic mobility in starch gels, due to amino acid substitutions which change the electric charge on the protein. Other variables include the isoelectric point, substrate affinity, response to inhibitors, pH optimum and temperature stability. Electrophoretic variants of human serum proteins have been extensively studied, and many allelic systems defined. Until DNA RFLPs were discovered, these were the main class of mendelian polymorphisms known. Protein polymorphisms give information only about expressed sequences, which may follow different evolutionary dynamics from the non-coding DNA where most RFLPs are found.

System	Locus symbol	Map location	Major antigens	Major alleles
ABO	ABO	9q34	A,B (A$_2$)	I^A,I^B,i
Rhesus	RH	1p36	C,c,D,E,e	CDE, CDe etc
Kell	KEL	?	K,k	K,k
P	P	6?	P$_1$,P$_2$	P$_1$,P$_2$,p
MNSs	MN	4q28–q31	M,N,S	MS,Ms, NS,Ns
Duffy	FY	1p21–q23	Fy^a,Fy^b	Fy^a,Fy^b,Fy
Kidd	JK	18(?)	Jk^a,Jk^b	Jk^a,Jk^b,Jk
Lutheran	LU	19p13–q13	Lu^a,Lu^b	Lua,Lub
Xg	XG	Xp22	Xg(a)	Xg(a+), Xg(a−)

Fig. 5.4 The main blood group systems.

Mendelian diseases follow the pedigree patterns of mendelian characters. Thousands of mendelian diseases are known, all individually rare but collectively they seriously affect 1% of newborns. No attempt is made here to list them all. For lists, brief descriptions and references, you should consult the successive editions of McKusick's 'Mendelian Inheritance in Man' (John Hopkins University Press, Baltimore, 8th edn 1988).

	Autosomal		X-linked
	Dominant	**Recessive**	
Pedigree pattern	vertical	horizontal	"knight's move"
Affects	both sexes	both sexes	mainly males
Parents	usually one affected	both usually unaffected	both usually unaffected
Risk to children	50%	small	50% for sons of carrier
Consanguinity	no	often	no
New mutations	frequent	rare	frequent
Variable expression	frequent	infrequent	in females
Example	fig 5-2b	fig 5-2c	fig 5-2f

Fig. 5.5 Main features of each mode of inheritance.

Autosomal dominant diseases affect heterozygotes. Homozygotes may be more severely affected than heterozygotes, as in achondroplasia, or indistinguishable, as in Huntington's disease. Homozygotes are seen only if two affected people marry, which with many rare or severe conditions has not been recorded.

Variable expression means the same gene causes symptoms varying in kind or severity in different people. This is a very common feature of dominant diseases. It can happen within families, and a minimally affected person can have a severely affected child, or vice versa. The geneticist must know the minimal signs of a disease, so that possible carriers can be examined for signs of the gene. Variable expression is seen whenever the effect of the main disease gene can be modulated by other genes or the environment.

Anticipation is the supposed tendency of dominant diseases to become more severe in succeeding generations. This does not really happen. The impression arises with diseases where severely affected people rarely reproduce. Families are ascertained through a severely affected child, and looking back through the pedigree, a parent and grandparent are seen to be mildly affected.

Disease	Locus symbol and chromosomal location		Incidence in UK
Huntington's disease	HD	4p16	1/20,000
Neurofibromatosis	NF1	17q12	1/ 3,000
Hypercholesterolaemia	FHC	19p13	1/ 500
Tuberous sclerosis	TS	9q34 (?)	1/30,000
Achondroplasia	ACH	?	1/25,000
Polycystic kidney disease	PKD1	16p13	1/ 1,000

Fig. 5.6 Examples of autosomal dominant diseases.

Dominant mutations. If a dominant condition prevents affected people from reproducing, then all cases must be fresh mutations. Many sporadic lethal conditions may be due to dominant mutations. With less serious conditions, the proportion of cases which are new mutations depends on the extent to which affected people reproduce. Formulae are given in Chapter 8.

Penetrance means the probability that a person carrying the gene for a dominant disease will manifest it. For a true dominant it should always be 100% but in fact different diseases have characteristically different penetrances. If the penetrance is too low, a disease is better treated as non-mendelian (*see* Chapter 7). Non-penetrance is a pitfall for genetic counselling. In Fig. 5.7, II_5 may carry the disease gene. The risk for III_4 is $p/2[(1-p)/(2-p)]$ if the penetrance is p. The maximum risk is 8.6% for $p = 0.6$.

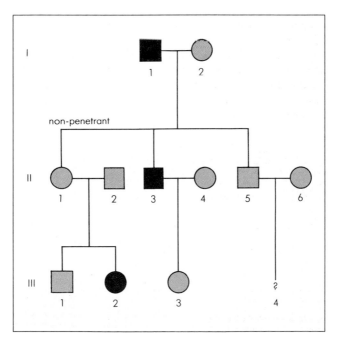

Fig. 5.7 Autosomal dominant pedigree with non-penetrance.

Late onset diseases include several dominant conditions. The gene is present at conception but clinical symptoms manifest only much later. Huntington's disease is a striking example. Before gene tracking was available, individuals such as III_1, in Fig. 5.8 had to decide whether to have children without knowing whether or not they carried the disease gene. Bayesian statistics is used to calculate risks in diseases with age-related penetrance (*see* Example 1, p.000).

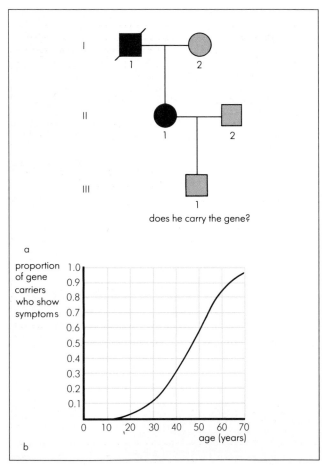

Fig. 5.8 Huntington's disease pedigree and onset curve.

X-linked recessive diseases are readily recognizable from the pedigree pattern (Fig. 5.2f). Male to male transmission does not occur because a father does not pass his X to his son.

New mutations are frequently the cause in serious conditions. With lethal diseases like Duchenne muscular dystrophy one affected male in three is believed to be a new mutant.

Disease	Locus symbol and chromosomal location		Incidence in UK (males)
Duchenne muscular dystrophy	DMD	Xp21	1/ 3,000
haemophilia A and B	F8C,F9	Xq27–q28	1/ 5,000
fragile-X mental retardation	FRAXA	Xq27	1/ 1,000
ectodermal dysplasia	EDA	Xq12	1/50,000
glucose 6 phosphate dehydrogenase deficiency	G6PD	Xq28	rare in UK

Fig. 5.9 Examples of X-linked recessive diseases.

Homozygotes, with an affected father and a carrier mother

Females with Turner syndrome

Carriers of X-autosome translocations (Chapter 4)

Manifesting heterozygotes

Fig. 5.10 Females affected with X-linked recessive conditions.

Boy mutant, mother not a carrier	1/3
Mother a carrier but grandmother not	1/3
Mother and grandmother both carriers	1/3

Fig. 5.11 New mutations in a lethal X-linked disease (assuming equal mutation rates in males and females).

Obligate carriers are females who have both a previous family history and an affected son or obligate carrier daughter. Women with two affected sons but no previous history are not obligate carriers because they may be germinal mosaics (*see* p. 103).

Manifesting heterozygotes are carrier women who show symptoms of an X-linked recessive disease, usually mild, because by bad luck they happen to have inactivated the normal X in most of the relevant cells.

Carrier testing relies on expression of the disease gene in cells where the normal X is inactivated, or within families on gene tracking. Carriers of glucose 6-phosphate dehydrogenase deficiency have a mixture of normal and deficient red cells; carriers of ectodermal dysplasia have patches of skin lacking sweat glands. Where the carrier test involves a diffusible product it is less reliable. Carriers of haemophilia often have lowered Factor VIII or IX levels, and carriers of Duchenne muscular dystrophy often have raised serum creatine kinase levels (by leakage from diseased muscle cells). These carrier tests give likelihoods which must be combined with the pedigree probability using Bayesian statistics.

X-linked dominant diseases give a much less recognizable

Disease	Locus symbol and chromosomal location		Incidence in UK
hypophosphataemia	HPDR	Xp22	1/20,000
conditions lethal in males:			
incontinentia pigmenti	IP	Xp11?	rare
focal dermal hypoplasia	FDH	X	rare
chondrodysplasia punctata	CDPX	Xp22?	rare

Fig. 5.12 Examples of X-linked dominant disease.

pedigree pattern (Fig. 5.2e). The pattern resembles an autosomal dominant pedigree except that all daughters but no sons
of an affected man are affected. Symptoms in females are
usually milder and more variable than in males because of
lyonization. The best proof of X-linkage is to demonstrate
linkage with known X-chromosome markers.

AUTOSOMAL RECESSIVE DISEASES

Autosomal recessive diseases affect only homozygotes, though
heterozygotes may be detectable biochemically. Fig. 5.2c
shows the pattern of inheritance. Cases are often sporadic with
no previous family history, but it is important to recognize the
inheritance because the recurrence risk is 1 in 4.

Consanguinity is measured by the coefficient of relationship of
the parents and the coefficient of inbreeding of the child (*see*
Chapter 8). The danger of inbreeding is often exaggerated. In
the UK the risk of a seriously abnormal child (all causes) is
about 2% for an unrelated couple and about 4% for first cousins.

Carrier testing is possible where heterozygotes have lowered
enzyme activity, or by gene tracking within families.

Disease	Locus symbol and chromosomal location		Incidence
cystic fibrosis	CF	7q22	1/2,000 (UK)
phenylketonuria	PKU	12q24.1	1/10,000 (UK)
sickle cell disease	HBB	11p15.5	1/100 (W.Africa)
alpha-thalassaemia	HBA	16p13	1/100 (Thailand)
beta-thalassaemia	HBB	11p15.5	1/100 (Sardinia)
adrenal hyperplasia	CAH1	6p21.3	1/10,000 (UK)

Fig. 5.13 Examples of autosomal recessive diseases.

Abnormalities	Mating	Offspring	Phenotype
Allelic	$a_1a_1 \times a_2a_2$	a_1a_2	Abnormal
Non-allelic	aaBB × AAbb	AaBb	Normal

Fig. 5.14 The complementation test.

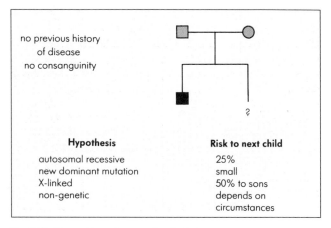

Hypothesis	Risk to next child
autosomal recessive	25%
new dominant mutation	small
X-linked	50% to sons
non-genetic	depends on circumstances

no previous history of disease
no consanguinity

Fig. 5.15 The problem of a sporadic affected case.

The complementation test shows whether two recessive (autosomal or X-linked) abnormalities are allelic. Two individuals, one with each abnormality, are mated. In humans of course such interesting matings rarely happen. Complementation has been observed in recessive deafness and in albinism, and can be studied where the phenotype is observable in cultured cells which can be fused *in vitro*.

DIFFICULTIES IN PEDIGREE INTERPRETATION

Sporadic cases. The questions to ask are
● is the condition recognizable as one with known cause (e.g. cystic fibrosis)?
● is there a likely environmental cause (e.g. drugs in pregnancy)?

Time	1966	1969	1988
Pedigree (no previous family history of this disease)	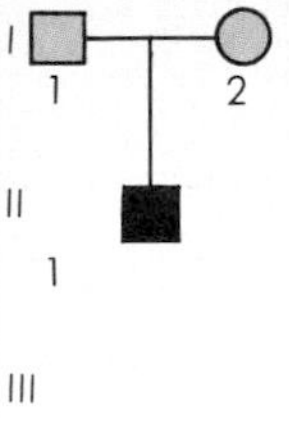	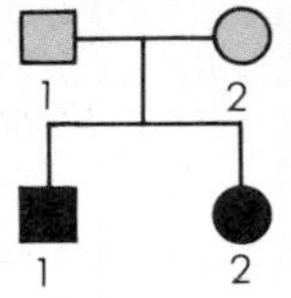	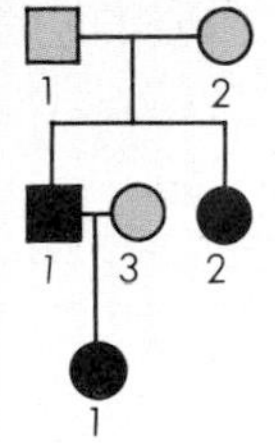
Postulated inheritance	dominant (new mutation)	recessive	dominant (germinal mosaic)
Risk of I_1 and I_2 having another affected child	very low	1 in 4	uncertain; up to 1 in 2
Risk of II_1 having an affected child	1 in 2	very low	1 in 2

Fig. 5.16 A misleading pedigree due to germinal mosaicism.

Germinal mosaicism means a person has two germ cell lines because of a mutation at some stage in development. If the mutation causes a dominant or X-linked recessive disease, a germinal mosaic can have two or more children each apparently carrying the disease as a fresh mutation. As Fig. 5.16 shows, this can lead to considerable problems in pedigree interpretation.

Gene tracking means using linked markers (usually RFLPs) to follow the transmission of a disease gene in a family. Gene tracking can be done only in families with a suitable pedigree structure. Several markers are needed so that if one marker is uninformative, another can be tried. This indirect method of following a disease gene would not be used where it is possible to test a person directly for the presence or absence of the disease mutation. Its value is for diseases where the map location is known but not the nature of the mutation.

Tracking using a single linked marker is illustrated by Figs 5.18 and 5.19. Note the requirement for a suitable pedigree structure in each case: in Fig. 5.18 the grandmother is needed and in Fig. 5.19 the affected child.

Recombination errors limit the accuracy of gene tracking. In Fig. 5.18 the prediction for III_1 is wrong if he is a recombinant. The probability of error equals the recombination fraction θ. In Fig. 5.19 the prediction will be wrong if recombination occurred in any of the four meioses producing the two offspring. In half the cases, however, a recombination error would make the fetus homozygous unaffected, so the risk of a false negative prediction with the results shown in Fig. 5.19 is 2θ.

1. Find a linked marker for which the person transmitting the disease is heterozygous, so that the two chromosomes can be told apart.

2. Establish phase, i.e. work out which marker allele is on the disease-bearing chromosome.

3. Work out which marker allele the consultand inherited.

Fig. 5.17 The three stages of gene tracking.

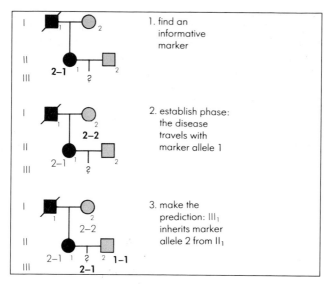

Fig. 5.18 Gene tracking in an autosomal dominant disease.

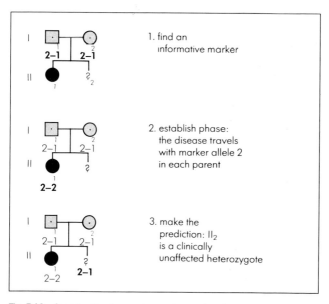

Fig. 5.19 Gene tracking in an autosomal recessive disease.

105

Bridging markers are pairs of linked markers, one mapping either side of the disease locus. If each marker shows 10% recombination with the disease locus, the prediction is wrong only if there is a double recombination. The chance of this is 10% of 10%, i.e. 1%.

Flanking markers is another term for bridging markers.

Intragenic RFLPs are used in gene tracking like linked RFLPs but with the advantage that recombination errors should be negligible.

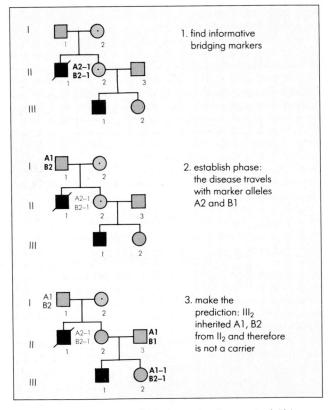

Fig. 5.20 Gene tracking in an X-linked recessive disease using bridging markers.

Bayesian statistics is a method of combining probabilities which is much used in estimating genetic risks. For example the risk that an asymptomatic person carries the gene for Huntington's disease is calculated by combining the mendelian risk from the pedigree with an age-related likelihood (the older an asymptomatic person is, the less likely they are to carry the disease gene), and maybe a likelihood derived from studies of linked RFLPs in the family.

The formal statement of Bayes's theorem is

$$P(H_i|E) = \frac{P(H_i)P(E|H_i)}{\sum P(H_i)P(E|H_i)}$$

$P(H_i)$ is the probability that hypothesis H_i is true (the prior probability)

$P(H_i|E)$ means the probability of H_i given observation E

$P(E|H_i)$ means the probability of observation E given that H_i is true (the conditional probability).

Example 1 What is the probability that the asymptomatic 45-year old son of a woman with Huntington's disease carries the disease gene?

Hypotheses: H_1: he does carry the HD gene
               H_2: he does not carry the gene

Prior probabilities (from mendelian genetics):
         $P(H_1) = 0.5$
         $P(H_2) = 0.5$
(note that the prior probabilities must sum to 1)

Conditional probabilities:
         $P(E|H_1) = 0.5$ (the probability that a 45-year old is asymptomatic given that he carries the HD gene, from Fig. 5.8)
         $P(E|H_2) = 1.0$ (he is certain to be asymptomatic on the hypothesis that he does not carry the HD gene)
(note that conditional probabilities do not necessarily sum to 1)

Bayesian calculation:

$$P(H_1|E) \ = \ \frac{0.5 \times 0.5}{(0.5 \times 0.5) + (0.5 \times 1.0)} \ = \ \frac{1}{3}$$

Thus his risk of carrying the gene has decreased from 1/2 at birth to 1/3 because he is still asymptomatic at age 45.

The calculation is usually set out like this:

hypothesis	carries HD	not carrier
prior risk	0.5	0.5
conditional risk: asymptomatic at age 45	0.5	1.0
joint risk (prior × conditionals)	0.25	0.5
final risk (joint/sum of joints)	$\frac{0.25}{0.75} = \frac{1}{3}$	$\frac{0.5}{0.75} = \frac{2}{3}$

Example 2 What is the risk a woman carries the Duchenne muscular dystrophy gene? Her mother was an obligate carrier but she has two normal sons and a low serum creatine kinase (CK) level: 70% of non-carriers but only 20% of carriers have a serum CK level this low.

hypothesis	carrier	not carrier
prior probability	0.5	0.5
conditionals:		
2 normal sons	0.25	1.0
low serum CK	0.20	0.70
joint:	0.025	0.35
overall carrier risk	0.025/0.375 = 0.066	

Note that any number of conditional probabilities can be included provided they are logically independent of one another.

6 | Biochemical Genetics

HAEMOGLOBINS AND HAEMOGLOBINOPATHIES

Gene clusters. All haemoglobins are coded by two gene clusters at chromosomal locations 16p13 and 11p15. In the alpha globin cluster two identical expressed genes are present on each chromosome, so that normal people have four functioning α-globin genes (Fig. 6.3). The non-alpha genes on chromosome 11 are all closely related structurally, but are expressed differently. In each cluster the genes at the 5' end are expressed earliest in embryogenesis, perhaps hinting at an unknown control mechanism.

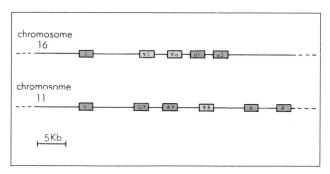

Fig. 6.1 The two globin gene clusters.

$\alpha_2\beta_2$	HbA	adult (major form)
$\alpha_2\delta_2$	HbA$_2$	adult (minor form)
$\alpha_2\gamma_2$	HbF	fetus
$\alpha_2\epsilon_2$	Hb Gower–2	embryo
$\zeta_2\gamma_2$	Hb Portland	embryo
$\zeta_2\epsilon_2$	Hb Gower–1	embryo

Fig. 6.2 Table of different haemoglobins.

Thalassaemias are caused by reduced (α^+ or β^+) or absent (α^0 or β^0) synthesis of the α or β globin chain. Both diseases affect millions of people worldwide and are associated with resistance to malaria. The molecular causes are extremely diverse and include gene deletions, mutations inactivating promoters, splice sites, polyadenylation signals and terminators, base changes causing premature termination and amino acid substitutions making the polypeptide unstable. Gene deletions are particularly frequent in α-thalassaemia, often in combination with chromosomes carrying a single α gene which arise by unequal recombination.

Variant haemoglobins. Over 200 structural variants have been described, mostly very rare, with amino acid substitutions caused by single base changes. Carriers may be normal or suffer from anaemia or other symptoms depending on how the function of the haemoglobin is affected. Three variants are common and are associated with resistance to malaria.

Hereditary persistence of fetal haemoglobin (HPFH) is a mendelian trait found in areas where β-thalassaemia or β structural variants are common. Clinically it often compensates for deficient β chain production or function. HPFH is

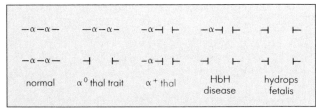

Fig. 6.3 Reduced α-globin gene dosage in α-thalassaemia.

HbS	β^6 glu → val	Africa, Mediterranean, Middle East
HbC	β^6 glu → lys	West Africa
HbE	β^{26} glu → lys	South-East Asia

Fig. 6.4 Common structural variants of haemoglobin.

usually caused by large deletions removing the δ and β genes; how these cause the HPFH phenotype is not known but the molecular cause is of interest for the light it should throw on developmental gene regulation.

Haplotypes in β-thalassaemia. β-globin clusters are classified by sequence framework and RFLP haplotypes. Each particular β-thalassaemia mutation tends to occur on one haplotype in a given population, reflecting the spread of ancestral mutants through the population. These associations are helpful for prenatal diagnosis: the mutation can be predicted from the haplotype, and an appropriate allele-specific probe used for diagnosis. Similar associations are seen in phenylketonuria and cystic fibrosis.

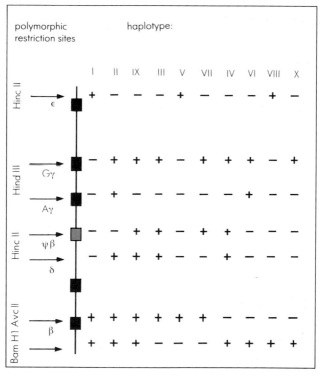

Fig. 6.5 Haplotypes associated with β-thalassaemia mutations.

Inborn errors of metabolism are caused by lack of activity of one specific enzyme in a metabolic pathway. Most are recessive (autosomal or occasionally X-linked) because one functioning copy of the gene is usually sufficient for normality.

Metabolic blocks cause deficiency of products beyond the block and accumulation of precursors. Either the deficiency or the accumulation may cause the clinical symptoms.

Lysosomal storage diseases exemplify inborn errors adequately well understood clinically and biochemically without the help of DNA technology. They are caused by lack of one or other of the degradative enzymes of the lysosome. High molecular weight material imported into lysosomes cannot be broken down or exported; it accumulates and eventually kills the cell. Affected children are normal at birth but the steady accumulation of material in lysosomes leads to progressive, usually lethal, degeneration.

Collagen disorders illustrate the difference between a clinical and a molecular classification of a group of diseases. Modes of inheritance and recurrence risks are being revised in the light of the molecular data.

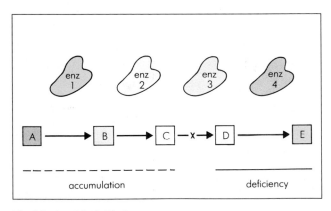

Fig. 6.6 A metabolic block.

Disease	Inheritance	Missing enzyme
mucopolysaccharidoses:		
Hunter syndrome	Xlr	iduronate sulphatase
Hurler syndrome	ar	α–L–iduronidase
sphingolipidoses:		
Niemann–Pick disease	ar	sphingomyelinase
Fabry disease	Xlr	α–galactosidase
Tay–Sachs disease	ar	hexosaminidase A
Gaucher disease	ar	β–glucosidase
mucolipidoses:		
I-cell disease	ar	many enzymes

Fig. 6.7 Examples of lysosomal storage diseases.

Clinical class and inheritance	Defective gene
osteogenesis imperfecta:	
type 1 (blue sclerae, Ad)	various defects in COL1A1 or COL1A2 in most cases. Disease phenotype depends on nature of mutation
type II (lethal perinatal, Ad)	
type III (severe deforming, ?Ar)	
type IV (mild, Ad)	
Ehlers–Danlos syndrome:	
type IV (fragile arteries, ?Ar)	COL3A1; in some cases COL1A1, COL1A2 or procollagen N-proteinase
type VII (short stature etc, ?Ad)	
Marfan syndrome (Ad)	?not collagen gene

Fig. 6.8 Examples of collagen disorders.

Phenylketonuria shows how a mendelian condition may be modified by the environment. Mental retardation can be avoided by screening children at birth and restricting dietary phenylalanine. Adult brains are not damaged by high phenylalanine levels, but treated women must go back on a low-phenylalanine diet during pregnancy otherwise the fetus (which is presumably heterozygous and therefore expected to be normal) suffers severe brain damage.

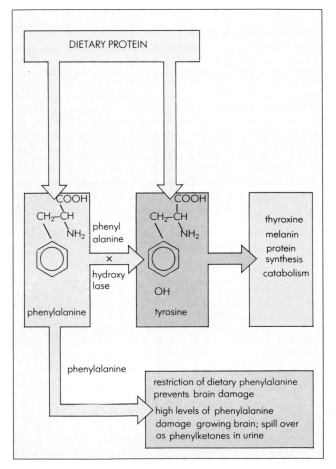

Fig. 6.9 Phenylketonuria.

Structure of antibody molecule always involves two identical heavy (H) chains of 450–600 amino acids and two identical light (L) chains of 230 amino acids, linked by disulphide bridges. H chains are of five main types, depending on the antibody class (γ, μ, δ, α, ε). L chains are of two types (κ, λ), each of which can be combined with any class of H chain. IgM and some IgA antibodies are polymers of this four-chain structure.

Isotypes are multiple forms of immunoglobulin molecules which coexist in normal individuals. Human isotypic variants include the heavy chain classes (γ, α, μ, δ, ε) and subclasses (IgG1, IgG2, IgG3, IgG4; IgA1, IgA2). Isotypes are not alleles: each has a separate gene (Fig. 6.14) and a normal person has all isotypes.

Allotypes are allelic variants of immunoglobulin molecules. The main allotypic systems are Gm, Am and Km (previously called Inv) which are located on the γ and α heavy chain and κ light chain respectively. Gm allotypes are divided into G1m, G2m and G3m systems, expressed on IgG1, IgG2 and IgG3 heavy chains, but some Gm antigens are common to several

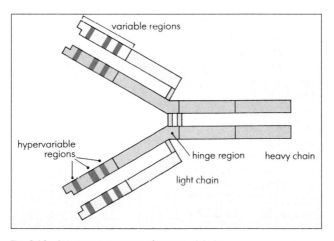

Fig. 6.10 Schematic structure of immunoglobulin.

classes (isoallotypes). A particular molecule may carry more than one antigen of an allotypic system, because amino acids at different positions in the chain are recognized by different antisera (just as a β-globin molecule could carry both the HbS and HbE variants, *see* Fig. 6.4). Each individual therefore has two Gm haplotypes each specifying a combination of Gm antigens, and these are useful polymorphic markers.

Idiotypes are the antigenic properties of individual immunoglobulin molecules. Each individual produces innumerable different idiotypes.

Variable (V) regions are the N-terminal 110 or so amino acids of H and L chains, which differ greatly among members of the same class within an individual. Most of the variability in V regions occurs in three hypervariable or complementarity determining regions (CDRs: amino acids 24–34, 50–56 and 89–97 of L chains, 31–35, 50–65, 95–102 of H chains), which are surrounded by relatively invariable framework (FR) regions. The CDRs are largely responsible for the antigen-binding specificity of an antibody.

Constant (C) regions show only allotypic or isotypic variation. They comprise one (L chains), three (γ, α, δ H chains) or four (μ, ε H chains) structural modules (domains). Each domain is coded by a separate exon of the corresponding gene.

Germ-line immunoglobulin genes comprise three complex loci. IGH at chromosomal location 14q32 encodes all heavy chains, IGK at 2p12 encodes κ light chains and IGL at 22qll encodes λ light chains. In each case sequences encoding the V and C regions are widely separated and up to several hundred V genes are present.

Joining (J) segments are DNA sequences encoding the dozen or so V-region amino acids adjoining the C region. 4–6 J region genes lie a few kilobases upstream of the C genes at each of the three loci.

Diversity (D) segments are found only in the IGH locus. They are a family of short DNA sequences located between the V and J genes or possibly among the V genes.

V–J and V–D–J splicing are a specialized form of recombination which is necessary before an immunoglobulin gene can be expressed. Splicing takes place during maturation of the B cell. As in meiotic recombination, DNA sequences are cut and joined, but in this case only one DNA strand is involved. A

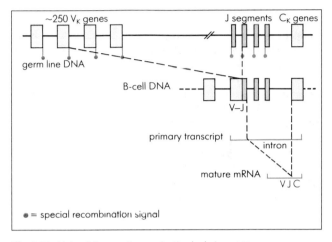

Fig. 6.11 V–J splicing creates productive L chain genes.

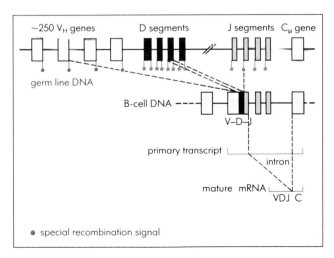

Fig. 6.12 V–D–J splicing creates productive H chain genes.

special enzyme system must be used for these recombinations which recognizes a specific signal sequence (● in Figs 6.11 and 6.12). Probably any one of the hundreds of V genes can be joined to any of the J segments. At the IGH locus a V gene is joined to a D segment, and a second recombination joins this to a J segment.

Variable position of recombination at the V–J boundary adds another layer of diversity by coding for different amino acids depending on the exact position of the V–J junction.

Somatic mutation occurs at the remarkably high rate of 10^{-3} mutations per base pair per cell generation in specific parts of all V genes (but at a negligible rate elsewhere). The mechanism is unknown, but the result is a large contribution to antibody diversity.

Membrane and secretory forms of heavy chains differ by having a transmembrane or a secretory signal polypeptide sequence at the C-terminal end. The mRNAs for the two forms are made by differential splicing of a single primary transcript which contains exons for both sequences.

Class switching. B cells initially produce IgM and/or IgD. Later they may switch to producing a different class of immunoglobulin, but still with the same idiotype and antigen specificity. Class switching requires another recombination event at the DNA level, in which the V–D–J sequence is brought into apposition to a new C sequence further downstream. This process does not use the special V–D–J recognition sequence. Recombination occurs in regions of tandem repeats (switch regions, *see* Fig. 6.14) which are located upstream of each C gene.

Allelic exclusion. Only one of the two homologous genes for each immunoglobin chain is expressed in each cell. Probably productive rearrangement of one gene inhibits rearrangement of its homologue. Alternatively, maybe most rearrangements are unsuccessful, so that a cell is unlikely to achieve productive rearrangement of both homologues.

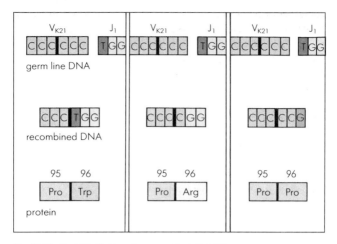

Fig. 6.13 Variable V–J junction generates diversity.

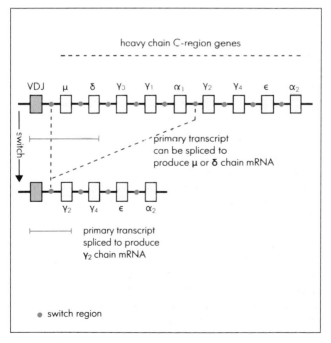

Fig. 6.14 Heavy chain class switching.

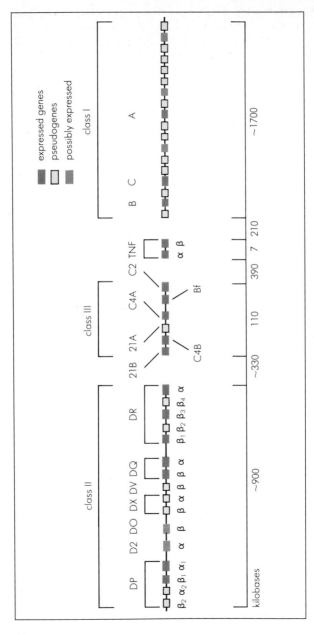

Fig. 6.15 The Major Histocompatibility Complex.

120

Major Histocompatibility Complex/System (MHC or MHS) is a 3.5 megabase region on the short arm of chromosome 6 which contains a cluster of genes mediating immune function and cell recognition: Class I and Class II HLA antigens, C2, C4 and Bf components of the complement system and tumour necrosis factor. The MHC also includes the structurally and functionally unrelated steroid 21-hydroxylase genes and probably the gene for idiopathic haemochromatosis. Linkage disequilibrium within the MHC is described in Chapter 7.

Class I antigens are cell surface antigens comprising highly polymorphic α-chains, coded within the MHC, complexed with the invariant β2-microglobulin which is coded by a gene on chromosome 15. In addition to the classical HLA A, B and C loci, about 20 other Class I genes are present. Many of these 'non-classical' Class I genes are pseudogenes, but some code for non-polymorphic antigens of unknown function. The Class I region also contains an unidentified gene which causes idiopathic haemochromatosis .

Class II antigens are cell surface molecules structurally and functionally closely related to Class I antigens. The polymorphic α and β chains are both encoded within the MHC and chains coded by different Class II loci can probably combine to form heterodimers.

Class III products (C2, C4, 21 hydroxylase, tumour necrosis factor) are unrelated to the Class I and II products. Two copies of the C4 and 21-OH genes are present because of a tandem duplication. The pairs retain over 98% DNA sequence homology and unequal recombination between them can produce chromosomes carrying one or three C4-21-OH pairs. The C4A, C4B and 21-OHB genes are functional but 21-OHA is a pseudogene.

Congenital adrenal hyperplasia (CAH) results from deficiency of 21-hydroxylase. The disturbed steroid metabolism virilizes females and aldosterone deficiency makes both sexes prone to life-threatening salt loss. 30% of the mutations are deletions of the functional 21-OHB gene. There is evidence of a high frequency of gene conversion (*see* Chapter 7) as well as point mutations and unequal recombination.

The immunoglobulin superfamily is a family of proteins each made of one or several domains having homology to either the V or C region immunoglobulin domains. Apart from the immunoglobulins themselves and the HLA Class I and II molecules, other members of the family include β_2-microglobulin, the T cell receptor chains and various lymphocyte surface proteins (CD3, CD4, CD8). Note however that the bewildering array of special genetic mechanisms which generate antibody diversity do not operate in any other members of the family except for the T cell receptor genes.

T-cell receptors are immunoglobulin-like molecules comprising two chains, each with constant and variable regions. There are four loci, coding for α, β, γ and δ chains, each of which is subject to rearrangements similar to those shown in Figs 6.11–6.13. Receptors comprising α/β and γ/δ dimers mark different subsets of T-cells, perhaps different developmental stages.

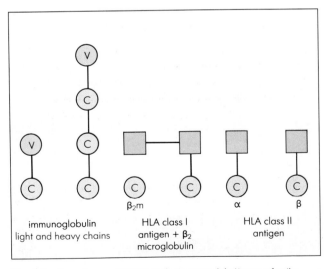

Fig. 6.16 Homologous domains in the immunoglobulin superfamily.

7 Non-mendelian Conditions

By far the greatest contribution of genetics to mortality and morbidity is through non-mendelian conditions.

There are many reasons why a character may be non-mendelian. In the past most genetic but non-mendelian traits were regarded as polygenic, but increasingly non-mendelian conditions are being approached analytically, looking for mendelian components.

Type of Genetic Abnormality		Frequency
Chromosomal		0.5%
Mendelian:	autosomal dominant	0.7%
	autosomal recessive	0.25%
	X-linked	0.05%
Non-mendelian:		
	congenital malformations	c.1%
	genetic factors in common diseases	c.5%

Fig. 7.1 Lifetime risk of serious genetic disease in UK.

Partially genetic characters:

- mendelian characters with environmental effects
- oligogenic characters with environmental effects
- polygenic characters with environmental effects

Genetic characters:

- quantitative characters
- heterogeneous characters
- oligogenic characters
- polygenic characters
- somatic characters

Fig. 7.2 Non-mendelian genetic characters.

Environment in the genetic sense means everything not genetic, including the intra-uterine environment.

Quantitative characters are characters which we all have, but to differing degrees, such as height, intelligence or tasting threshold for phenylthiocarbamide (PTC). If the distribution is bimodal, people can be classified as 'high' and 'low' and the difference tested for mendelian segregation, as with PTC tasting. When the population distribution is unimodal it is not possible to analyse the data in terms of segregating mendelian A and a alleles.

Discontinuous non-mendelian characters resemble mendelian characters in that people either have them or do not, but they do not show any of the characteristic mendelian segregation patterns in pedigrees. Examples are legion, including most common birth defects, the major psychoses and many common diseases of adult life.

Oligogenic characters are governed by a few (perhaps 2–5) loci. Rhesus haemolytic disease of the newborn happens when a Rh-ve mother carries an ABO-compatible Rh+ve fetus and the mother has been previously sensitized to Rh+ve red cells. If we did not understand the mechanism we would view it as a non-mendelian condition. Probably many non-mendelian conditions will appear equally simple in retrospect.

Heterogeneity is especially likely when the character being observed is the result of a long chain of events rather than the primary result of gene action. Childhood deafness for example is non-mendelian when viewed in aggregate, but it has many different causes, some purely environmental, some mendelian, and perhaps some truly non-mendelian.

Multifactorial is a catch-all term for conditions determined by a large number of genetic factors, with or without environmental contributions. Multifactorial theory means polygenic theory.

Non-genetic:	
congenital rubella	12
congenital cytomegalovirus	3
perinatal events	15
postnatal (meningitis etc)	5
Genetic:	
mendelian, dominant	13
mendelian, recessive	12
mendelian, mode not clear	3
chromosomal	5
Possibly genetic:	
congenital malformations	3
unknown (probably mostly recessive)	40

Fig. 7.3 A study of deafness in 111 Manchester children, showing heterogeneity.

IS IT GENETIC?

Mendelian and chromosomal conditions are self-evidently genetic, but for non-mendelian characters any genetic determination needs to be proved. The main methods are family correlations, twin concordance and adoption studies.

Family correlations measure the resemblance between relatives. For quantitative characters the correlation is rh^2, where r is the coefficient of relationship and h^2 the heritability. For discontinuous characters the incidence among relatives of an affected proband is compared to the population incidence.

Since humans give their children both their genes and their environment, claims for genetic determination based solely on family resemblance must be treated with great suspicion.

Monozygotic (MZ) twins derive from a single zygote. MZ twins are genetically identical clones.

Dizygotic (DZ) twins derive from two ova fertilized by different sperm. DZ twins have half their genes in common, on average and may be like-sex or unlike-sex. The proportion of all twin pairs who are DZ is approximately twice the proportion of unlike-sex pairs.

Zygosity determination was traditionally based on the fetal membranes (all monochorionic twins are MZ; dichorionic twins may be MZ or DZ) or blood grouping. Nowadays DNA fingerprinting (*see* Chapter 1) is the method of choice.

Twin studies compare the similarity of monozygotic and dizygotic twin pairs for the trait in question. On the assumption that twins of either sort have an equal degree of common environment, greater resemblance of MZ twins points to genetic effects. The main problems are getting sufficient numbers to work on uncommon conditions and avoiding biased ascertainment (strikingly similar pairs are more likely to be noticed). The result is expressed as the concordance, or for quantitative characters as the H statistic:

$$H = \frac{V_{DZ} - V_{MZ}}{V_{DZ}}$$ (V_{DZ} and V_{MZ} are the mean square differences within DZ and MZ pairs respectively)

Concordant twin pairs are both affected or both unaffected. Pairs where one is affected and the other unaffected are discordant.

Separated MZ twins should mean twins separated at birth and brought up with no contact. Resemblances between them are almost certain to be genetic. In practice reported series often include twins separated later or brought up by relatives. Even

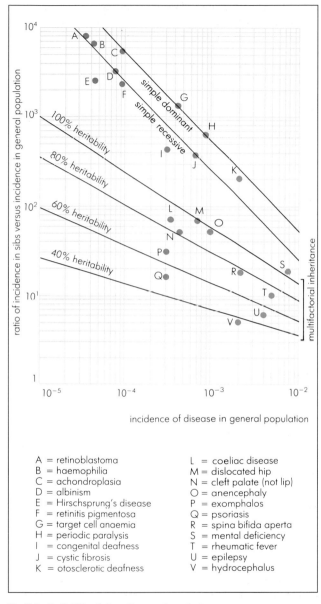

Fig. 7.4 Heritability of discontinuous characters.

twins separated at birth shared the intra-uterine environment.

Adoption studies are the most powerful tool for investigating genetic determination in conditions likely to depend on family environment e.g. schizophrenia. They are of two kinds:
- adoptees with the disease of interest are matched with healthy control adoptees, and the incidence of the disease in their biological and adoptive relatives is compared.
- probands with the disease are identified whose children were adopted away, and matched with unaffected parents whose children were also adopted away. The incidence of disease in the two groups of children is compared.

DISEASE ASSOCIATIONS AND LINKAGE DISEQUILIBRIUM

Relative risk (RR) of a disease, given marker type A, is

		type A	not A
RR = ad/bc	affected	a	b
	not affected	c	d

Disease associations. An allele or phenotype is associated with susceptibility (or resistance) to a disease if the RR is significantly different from unity. Note that while linkage is a relation between loci, associations are relations between alleles or phenotypes, e.g. ankylosing spondylitis is associated with HLA-B27, not with the HLA-B locus. A strong association points to a major genetic determinant. Associations between diseases and particular HLA types have been studied intensively in the hope of discovering major susceptibility genes, particularly for autoimmune diseases.

Disease-marker associations occur if the marker is in linkage disequilibrium with a disease susceptibility gene, if the marker itself confers susceptibility, or if there is population stratification. The association of HLA-B27 with ankylosing spondylitis may be because B27 cross-reacts with a bacterial antigen, leading to an abnormal immune response. HLA-DR3 and DR4 are probably associated with insulin-dependent diabetes because they are in disequilibrium with DQβ chains carrying an epitope which confers susceptibility. The existence of a strong population association, provided stratification has been ruled out as the cause, proves that a disease is not truly polygenic.

Linkage disequilibrium is a non-random association between particular alleles at two closely linked loci. It is seen with some, but by no means all, closely linked pairs of loci; the classic

Disease	Marker	% positive		RR
		Patients	Controls	
ankylosing spondylitis	B27	90	9	82
rheumatoid arthritis	DR4	58	25	4.1
insulin-dependent				
diabetes	DR3	46	22	3.1
	DR4	51	25	3.1
narcolepsy	DR2	100	31	–
gluten-sensitive				
enteropathy	DPα RFLP	78	35	6.6

Fig. 7.5 Examples of HLA-disease associations.

antigen 1 freq = p_1		antigen 2 freq = p_2		haplotype 1,2		
				obs	exp (p_1p_2)	Δ
HLA-A1	.138	HLA-B8	.090	.0609	.0124	+0.491
HLA-A1	.138	HLA-B7	.098	.0044	.0135	−0.089
HLA-B8	.090	HLA-DR3	.118	.074	.0106	+0.686

Fig. 7.6 Examples of linkage disequilibrium in the MHC.

examples are in the MHC. It is measured by the gametic associaion or standardized disequilibrium coefficient.

Gametic association is $D = ad - bc$

Standardized disequilibrium coefficient is

$$\Delta = \frac{ad-bc}{\sqrt{(a+c)(b+d)(a+b)(c+d)}}$$

where a, b, c, d are the frequencies of the haplotypes A1B1, A1B2, A2B1 and A2B2 respectively.

Linkage does not in itself produce associations. Considering loci A and B, if the A2 allele first appeared as a mutation on a chromosome carrying B1, the initial association between A2 and B1 would be gradually broken up by recombination. Each generation the gametic association D decreases by a factor 1-r where r is the recombination rate. For $r = 0.01$, D will be halved in 70 generations or less than 2000 years ($0.99^{70} = 0.49$). Thus without selection linkage disequilibrium should be seen only for very closely linked loci and recent mutations. Long persisting disequilibrium must be due to selection for or against particular haplotypes. The reasons for the strong associations seen in the major histocompatibility complex are unknown.

Stratification means the population studied consists of two or more reproductively isolated groups. A non-genetic association arises if most cases of the disease occur in one group which happens to have a high frequency of some marker. Sib-pair analysis (*see* Chapter 3) would show no association.

Recurrence risks in multifactorial disorders are empiric risks, i.e. they are estimated from survey data not from theory. Polygenic theory does suggest a few generalizations:
• the recurrence risk increases with the number of previously affected children. This is quite different from mendelian recurrence risks, which are independent of family history once the genotypes have been identified. It is not, of course, that having another affected child causes the risk to go up,

	Cleft lip +/− palate	Pyloric stenosis		Neural tube defect
Population incidence	1/1000	5/1000 (males)	1/1000 (females)	3/1000
Incidence among relatives:				
1st degree	×40	×10–25	×30–50	×15
2nd degree	× 7	× 5	× 5	× 5
3rd degree	× 2–3	× 2	× 2	× 2
Heritability	80%	80%	90%	80%

Fig. 7.7 Empiric risks (these risks are for illustration only and should not be used for counselling).

rather it permits identification of the high risk which was always present.

- where there is a sex difference in incidence of the condition, the recurrence risk is greater after the birth of an affected child of the rarer sex.
- the risk is highest for monozygotic co-twins, and decreases through first and second degree relatives, to near the population level with third degree relatives.
- if the population incidence is q, the risk to first degree relatives is approximately $\sqrt{q}$.

POLYGENIC THEORY

Polygenic theory assumes that a trait is governed by the action of a large number of separate gene loci, each of individually small effect. As always when the outcome depends on a large number of independent small causes, the phenotype shows a gaussian distribution defined by its mean and variance (or standard deviation). The variance can be partitioned into components by standard statistical methods:

$$V_P = V_G + V_E$$

V_P = total variance of phenotype

V_G = phenotypic variance due to genetic differences

V_E = phenotypic variance due to environmental differences

The genetic variance can be further partitioned:

$$V_G = V_A + V_D$$

V_A = additive genetic variance

V_D = dominance variance

Polygenic conditions are often impossible to prove, because the data fit equally well the predictions of polygenic and of single major locus models. Thus the most useful line of research is to try to show that a condition is *not* polygenic, by looking for major environmental determinants, heterogeneity, associations with markers and indications of linkage.

Additive variance measures all genetic effects except those caused by particular combinations of genes, and is much the largest component of genetic variance.

Dominance variance. Dominance introduces a small extra variance because the phenotypic effect of a gene depends on the combination of alleles at a locus.

Interaction variances allow for interactions between genes and environment. For example it is supposed that high IQ parents give their children not just high IQ genes but also an environment conducive to development of the intellect. This requires an interaction variance

$$V_P = V_A + V_D + V_E + V_I$$

Each additional parameter makes it harder to estimate any one value from experimental data, and investigations of the genetics of IQ tend to founder in a sea of parameters even if they pass the initial hurdle of agreeing what to measure.

Degree of genetic determination or **broad heritability** is V_G/V_P.

Heritability (h^2) is defined as V_A/V_P. The degree to which a population can be changed by selective breeding is a function of h^2, not of the broad heritability. h^2 varies between 0 (purely environmental) and 1 (purely genetic). High heritability means that most of the reason why some people get a disease while others do not is because of the genetic differences between them. It does not mean the disease is untreatable but it does mean that the range of environments common in that population have little effect. In a population with a wider range of environments the heritability might be lower.

Regression to the mean has been the subject of more myths and fallacies than any other topic in genetics. The simple model in Fig. 7.8 illustrates how it works. Three major fallacies are as follows:
- after a few generations everybody will be exactly the same. In Fig. 7.8 the average for the children of each class of father is halfway between the father's score and the population mean, but the overall distribution in the children is the same as in the fathers. Regression works both ways: the average for the fathers of each class of children is halfway between the children's score and the population mean.
- the average for the children is halfway between the population mean and the average of the two parents. This would be true only if the variance were entirely due to dominance and epistasis, a most unlikely circumstance. The average for the children is where common sense says it should be, the same as the average of the parents. If there is random mating, then the average for the children will indeed be halfway between the score of one parent and the population mean; this is because with random mating the average score for the other parent equals the population mean.
- regression to the mean is evidence of a genetic mechanism. It

will occur whenever parent and child share some but not all of the determinants of their phenotype. The determinants can be environmental or genetic.

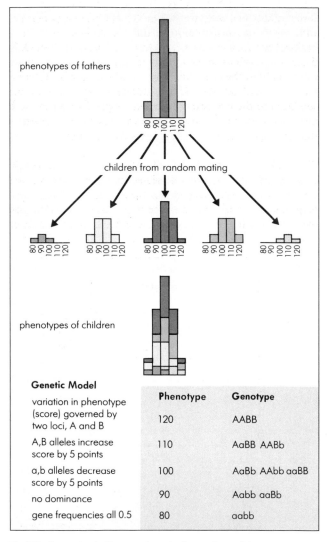

Genetic Model		
variation in phenotype (score) governed by two loci, A and B	**Phenotype**	**Genotype**
	120	AABB
A,B alleles increase score by 5 points	110	AaBB AABb
a,b alleles decrease score by 5 points	100	AaBb AAbb aaBB
no dominance	90	Aabb aaBb
gene frequencies all 0.5	80	aabb

Fig. 7.8 Regression to the mean in a simple genetic model.

One theory of discontinuous non-mendelian characters is that there is an underlying genetic susceptibility or liability. Everybody has susceptibility, but some people have high susceptibility and others low. The susceptibility is polygenic, with a gaussian distribution in the population, and with a heritability which can be estimated from family studies. Only those people whose susceptibility exceeds a certain threshold value manifest the character. The threshold may be different for males and females, giving different incidences of the condition in the two sexes. Affected people share genes with their relatives, so the distribution of liability in relatives is shifted upwards compared to the general population.

Cleft palate is a good example of a polygenic threshold condition. In the embryo the palatal shelves are separate and vertical. Within the appropriate time in the developmental program they must become horizontal and fuse. Provided they do fuse, it does not matter whether they fuse early or

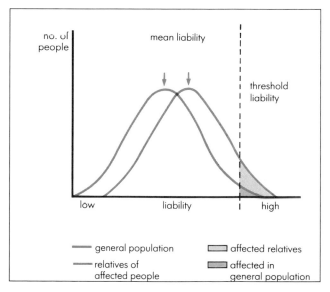

Fig. 7.9 Distribution of liability.

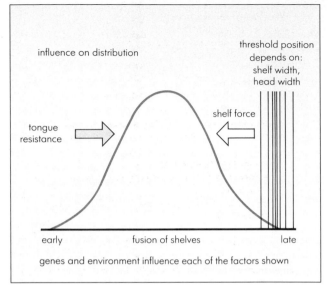

Fig. 7.10 Multifactorial cleft palate.

late, but if they miss, the result is cleft palate. Susceptibility is truly polygenic: many genetic and environmental factors affect the stage at which the shelves become horizontal. The position of the threshold also depends on the relative widths of the head and the palatal shelves. Nevertheless, in individual cases single major causes may predominate, so that in addition to the polygenic-threshold cleft palates there are mendelian and chromosomal cleft palates.

SOMATIC CONDITIONS

Somatic conditions are due to genetic changes in only certain cells in the body. In all normal mendelian and non-mendelian conditions we assume the genotype in question was present in the original fertilized egg and is found in all cells of the body. The ability to study human genes biochemically in cell cultures, rather than just follow pedigree patterns, has opened the way to a whole new area of genetics: conditions caused by genetic changes in somatic cells.

Chromosomal mosaics (Chapter 4):
mosaic Down's syndrome etc
mosaics for karyotypes lethal in non-mosaic form
chromatid abnormalities

Genetic mosaics:
females heterozygous for X-linked conditions
germinal mosaics in Duchenne dystrophy etc
syndromes with skin markings following Blaschko's lines
syndromes with asymmetry or patchy tissue distribution

probably all cancers, especially:
hereditary cancers, with loss of heterozygosity:
retinoblastoma (13q14)
WAGR (Wilms tumour – aniridia – genital abnormalities) complex, 11p13
bilateral acoustic neuroma (22q)
familial adenomatous polyposis (5q21–q22)

non-hereditary tumours with type-specific genetic changes:
specific loss of heterozygosity:
5q markers in colorectal cancer
3p21 markers in lung and other cancers
specific chromosome abnormalities (fig.4-19)

Fig. 7.11 Somatic genetic conditions.

Loss of heterozygosity means finding that tumour tissue is homozygous for a marker for which the other tissue of the patient is heterozygous. Consistent and tumour-specific loss of a particular marker implies a retinoblastoma-like mechanism (Fig. 7.12) and pinpoints the location of the gene responsible.

Retinoblastoma is a malignant tumour of the eye, which can be unilateral or bilateral. It occurs sporadically or as an autosomal dominant condition. This rare disease is the model for a whole class of somatic conditions. At the cellular level retinoblastoma is recessive: neoplasia occurs in retinal cells having lost both copies of an anti-oncogene at chromosomal location 13q14.

In familial retinoblastoma the inherited abnormality is the loss of one functional gene, usually by a chromosome microdeletion. A somatic mutation inactivates the remaining functional gene, converting a cell to the tumour phenotype. Given the number of target cells, it is probable that such a mutation will occur in at least one cell. Thus at the pedigree level we see an autosomal dominant susceptibility mapping to 13q14, producing unilateral or bilateral disease. A variety of mechanisms have been shown to cause loss of the second gene in familial retinoblastoma.

Two-hit mechanism means two independent mutations are needed to cause the disease, as in retinoblastoma. Two-hit mechanisms explain why somatic diseases can run in families.

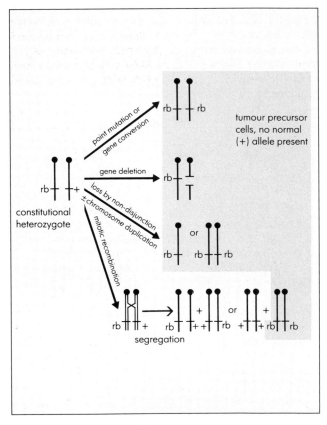

Fig. 7.12 Mechanisms in retinoblastoma.

Mitotic recombination is an abnormal event which can lead to loss of heterozygosity for markers distal to the crossover.

Gene conversion is the replacement of one allele at a locus by a copy of another allele which is present elsewhere in the cell, either on the homologous chromosome or another copy on the same chromosome. Gene conversion may be common in man, but the result is rarely distinguishable from the result of recombination or mutation.

Blaschko's lines map clonal boundaries in the skin. Chromosomal mosaics occasionally show patchy depigmentation following Blaschko's lines (hypomelanosis of Ito). Female carriers of X-linked skin conditions have patches of normal and abnormal skin following these lines, which mark boundaries between clones with different lyonization patterns. Skin markings following Blaschko's lines point to the presence of two different cell lines, often indicating a somatic genetic condition.

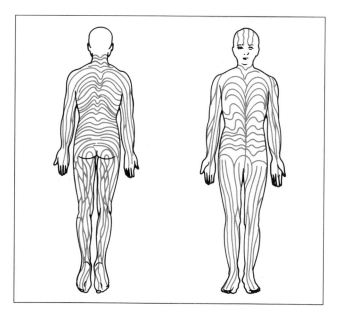

Fig. 7.13 Blaschko's lines.

8 | Genes in Populations

The **gene frequency** of allele A_1 is the chance that an allele at that locus, picked at random from the population, is A_1. It is also the proportion of all alleles at that locus which are A_1. Gene frequencies are conventionally symbolized by p or q and lie in the range 0–1.

Hardy–Weinberg distribution relates the frequencies of genotypes in a population to the gene frequencies. It is seen whenever the products of random mating are counted in an unbiased way.

This holds whether or not $p+q=1$ (i.e. whether or not A_1 and A_2 are the only alleles at the locus). For ABO blood groups, if the gene frequencies of the I^A, I^B and i genes are q_1, q_2 and q_3 respectively, the expected genotype frequencies are shown in Fig. 8.2.

Genotype	A_1A_1	A_1A_2	A_2A_2
Frequency	p^2	$2pq$	q^2

Fig. 8.1 Genotype frequencies from a Hardy–Weinberg distribution where alleles A_1 and A_2 have frequencies p and q.

Phenotype	A		B		AB	O
Genotype	I^AI^A	I^Ai	I^BI^B	I^Bi	I^AI^B	ii
Frequency	q_1^2	$2q_1q_3$	q_2^2	$2q_2q_3$	$2q_1q_2$	q_3^2

Fig. 8.2 Expected genotype frequencies for ABO blood groups.

For an X-linked character with alleles A_1 and A_2 with frequencies p and q, the genotype frequencies are shown in Fig. 8.3.

The Hardy–Weinberg distribution is easily understood by imagining you pick two genes at random from the population. The chance the first one is A_1 is p. The chance the second one is A_1 is also p. The chance that both are A_1 is therefore p^2. The chance of picking first A_1 then A_2 is pq, and the chance of picking first A_2 then A_1 is also pq. Thus the chance of picking one A_1 and one A_2 is 2pq.

Deviations from the Hardy–Weinberg distribution are seen whenever the analogy given above of picking genes at random from the population does not hold. Inbreeding and population stratification are the main causes. Deviations are also seen if there is selective gain or loss of a particular genotype (e.g. by natural selection or migration) in one generation before it is counted.

Random mating means that the probability of individual A selecting individual B as his mate does not depend on the genotype of B. Mating is random or non-random for a particular locus, e.g. mating is random for ABO blood group because nobody demands to know someone's blood group before deciding whether or not to marry.

Assortative mating is non-random mating. It can be either a tendency of like to marry like or of opposites to marry. Mating is assortative for height, build, intelligence, and also for some

	Males		Females		
Genotype	A_1	A_2	A_1A_1	A_1A_2	A_2A_2
Frequency	p	q	p^2	2pq	q^2

Fig. 8.3 Genotype frequencies for an X-linked character.

Phenotype	unaffected		affected
Genotype	AA	Aa	aa
Frequency	p^2	$2pq$	$q^2 = 1/10,000$

$q^2 = 1/10,000$ therefore $q = 1/100$ therefore $p = 99/100$

carrier frequency $= 2pq = 2 \times 99/100 \times 1/100 \simeq 1/50$

Fig. 8.4 Carrier frequencies for recessive conditions.

diseases such as deafness and achondroplasia. Assortative mating on any significant scale results in a non-Hardy–Weinberg distribution of genotypes in the progeny.

Carrier frequencies for recessive conditions are estimated on the assumption that the genotypes are in Hardy–Weinberg distribution. If the incidence of an autosomal recessive disease is known we can estimate the carrier frequency (Fig. 8.4). This estimate will be incorrect if the genotypes are not in a Hardy–Weinberg distribution. In particular, if most affected people are the product of consanguineous marriages, this calculation will seriously over-estimate the frequency of carriers in the general population.

MUTATION RATES

Mutation rates are defined as the chance of the mutation occurring to one gene in one generation. Typical human mutation rates are 10^{-5}–10^{-6}. The Duchenne muscular dystrophy gene has the highest mutation rate of any adequately studied human gene, at 10^{-4} mutations of normal to disease allele per gene per generation.

autosomal dominant	$\mu = 1/2\, F(1-f)$	or	$\mu = sp$
autosomal recessive	$\mu = F(1-f)$	or	$\mu = sq^2$
X-linked recessive	$\mu = 1/3\, F(1-f)$	or	$\mu = 1/3\, sq$

μ	= mutation rate per gene per generation
F	= incidence of condition
f	= biological fitness of affected people
s	= coefficient of selection
p,q	= frequencies of gene for dominant and recessive character respectively

Fig. 8.5 Indirect estimation of mutation rates.

Direct estimation of mutation rates for autosomal dominant conditions relies on simply counting the number of cases with unaffected parents. If 8 out of 100,000 consecutive newborns has a dominant condition and neither parent is affected, then 8 of the 200,000 genes have mutated. This method is extremely unreliable because of the likelihood of non-penetrance, non-paternity and failure to distinguish cases with recessive inheritance. All it can do is set a maximum mutation rate; the true rate will probably be much lower.

Indirect estimation of mutation rates relies on equations relating mutation rates to the frequency and severity of the condition.

These equations are based on several assumptions:
• there is equilibrium between the rate at which mutation creates disease genes and the rate at which selection removes them
• the mutation rate is the same in males and females
• there is random mating, giving a Hardy–Weinberg distribution of genotypes
• in recessive conditions, there is no selection in favour of heterozygotes. This is a potentially serious source of error.

143

Incidence of a condition is the proportion of a birth cohort who will have the condition at some time in their life.

Prevalence of a condition is the proportion of a surveyed population who have the condition at that time. Prevalences are usually lower than incidences because some affected cases may have already died, or people who carry the gene may not yet have developed the condition.

Biological fitness (f) of a genotype or phenotype is the average number of offspring produced by that type compared with the fittest type (or often, compared with the population average). f varies between 0 and 1. This genetic fitness may be very different from fitness in the conventional sense: a virilized female champion athlete may have zero fitness, while people with Huntington's chorea have been supposed to have higher fitness than their unaffected relatives.

Coefficient of selection (s) against a phenotype is the loss in biological fitness of that type compared to the standard normal type, i.e. $s = 1 - f$. A mutant persists in a large population for an average $1/s$ generations before being eliminated by selection.

Polymorphism is the existence of two or more alleles at significant frequencies in a population. A system is usually called polymorphic if more than one allele has a frequency of over 0.01.

Balanced polymorphism is a polymorphism where two or more alleles occur at frequencies too high to be maintained by recurrent mutation. The usual cause is selection in favour of the heterozygote. For example heterozygotes for sickle cell disease resist falciparum malaria better than normal homozygotes. The equilibrium frequency of the sickle gene is $s/(1+s)$, so the selection coefficient can be calculated from the gene frequency in a population. Selection in favour of the heterozygote probably underlies the high frequency of cystic fibrosis in Caucasians. The nature of the advantage is unknown.

Neutral polymorphisms are polymorphisms with no selective advantage or disadvantage to the different alleles. It is hard to be sure that any polymorphism really is neutral, but RFLPs in non-coding sequences seem good candidates.

Eugenics is the attempt to improve the genetic structure of the population by selective breeding. Negative eugenics means preventing or dissuading 'inferior' types from breeding; positive eugenics means persuading 'superior' types to have more children than average. Curiously, proponents of positive eugenics seem always to define their 'superior' type as persons like themselves. Eugenics has a bad name, and clinical geneticists are concerned to ensure that genetic counselling is not seen as part of any eugenic programme.

Eliminating genetic diseases by dissuading or preventing affected people from reproducing is a common idea among laymen. Unfortunately or otherwise, it usually won't work. Recessive diseases are maintained by a pool of carriers and preventing affected people from reproducing has little effect

Genotype	AA	AS	SS
Phenotype	normal	sickling trait	sickle cell disease
Fitness	$1-s$	1	0 (in the past)

Fig. 8.6 Sickle cell disease as a balanced polymorphism.

initial gene frequency q^0	.1	.01	.001	.0001
generations to halve it	10	100	1000	10,000

Fig. 8.7 Selection against a recessive disease.

(Fig. 8.7). Ignoring mutation, the gene frequency q_n after n generations of preventing affected people from reproducing is

$$q_n = q_o / (1 + n q_o)$$

where q_o is the original gene frequency. Sterilizing all carriers would be effective, but everybody carries several lethal recessive conditions.

If a dominant disease is serious enough to impair fertility, then most affected cases are new mutants and not preventable by eugenic measures. However, a program of prenatal diagnosis and abortion of affected fetuses could significantly reduce the frequency of serious late-onset dominants like Huntington's disease.

INBREEDING

Inbreeding means marrying relatives. In principle we are all related: Fig. 8.8 shows that if you were perfectly outbred the number of your ancestors would exceed the population of England 20 generations ago. Inbreeding is used to mean an unusually close relationship between spouses.

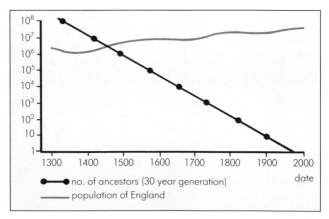

Fig. 8.8 The number of a person's ancestors.

146

Coefficient of inbreeding (F) is the probability that an individual receives at a given locus two genes which are identical by descent. The identity must be by descent from an ancestor common to both parents. F can be calculated from a pedigree by tracing all possible paths from one parent through each common ancestor and back to the other parent. Each path of n steps contributes $(1/2)^{n+1}$ to F (Fig. 8.10). This is Sewall Wright's path coefficient method.

Coefficient of kinship of two people is the probability that a gene taken at random from a locus in one person will be identical by descent to a gene taken at random from the same locus in the other person. It equals the coefficient of inbreeding of their offspring.

Coefficient of relationship (r) of two people is the proportion of their genes they share. Confusingly, r is twice the coefficient of kinship: if Fred is A1A2 and Jim is A1A3 at a locus, A1

Relation	Coefficient of relationship r	Coefficient of inbreeding of their offspring F
MZ twin	1	(MZ twins same sex)
first-degree relatives:		
DZ twin		
sib	0.5	0.25
parent		
child		
second-degree relatives:		
half-sib		
grandparent		
grandchild	0.25	0.125
uncle		
niece		
third-degree relatives:		
first cousin	0.125	0.0625

Fig. 8.9 Coefficients of relationship and inbreeding.

being identical by descent, they share half their genes, but there is only one chance in four of picking A1 from both Fred and Jim.

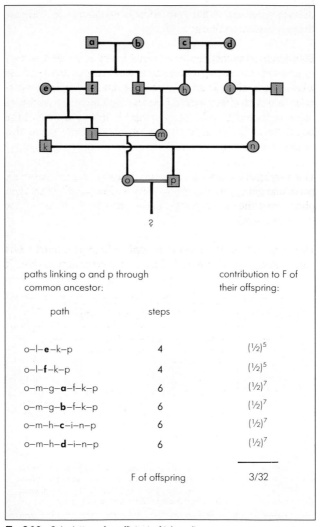

Fig. 8.10 Calculation of coefficient of inbreeding.

Segregation analysis compares the observed proportion of phenotypes among sibs or offspring with the segregation ratio predicted by a genetic hypothesis. The observed proportions must be corrected statistically for any bias of ascertainment. What correction is necessary depends on the mode of ascertainment.

Bias of ascertainment occurs when the sample of families used to estimate the segregation ratio is not representative of the whole population. It arises when the study sample is ascertained through affected people (as usually happens in studies of diseases) rather than by genotyping a random sample of the population. Different methods of ascertainment produce different biases.

The segregation ratio is the probability of a child having a particular gene, genotype or phenotype. For simple mendelian phenotypes the expected segregation ratio is 0.5 (dominant) or 0.25 (recessive).

The proband is the person through whom the family was ascertained (e.g. an affected child). In segregation analysis it

Ascertainment	Circumstances and correction
truncate	all families with any affected children ascertained — result of a thorough population survey. Correct by Li–Mantel method.
single	the probability a family is ascertained is proportional to the number of affected members — happens if a random small sample of all the cases in the population is studied, e.g. the first 100 patients at a clinic. Correct by sib method.
multiple	intermediate between single and truncate ascertainment — happens if condition is variable and mildly affected people get missed, or severely affected ones have already died. Correction is complex.

Fig. 8.11 Three ways of ascertaining families with a disease.

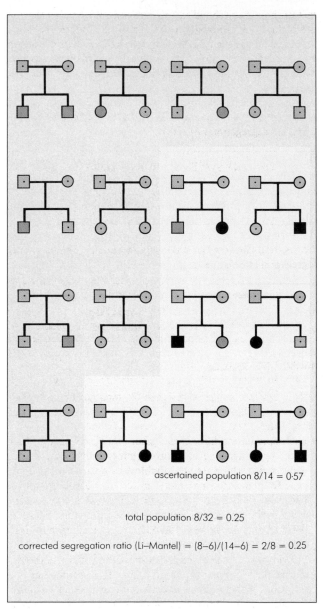

ascertained population 8/14 = 0·57

total population 8/32 = 0.25

corrected segregation ratio (Li–Mantel) = (8–6)/(14–6) = 2/8 = 0.25

Fig. 8.12 Truncate ascertainment.

matters how the proband was ascertained, and whether there is more than one proband in the family (i.e. more than one independent ascertainment). For counselling, the perceptions and needs of the proband and his close relatives may be different from those of more distant relatives, even if the risk is the same.

Li–Mantel method corrects for truncate ascertainment. The corrected segregation ratio is:

$$p = (R - S) / (T - S)$$

T = total individuals
R = total affected
S = total affected with no affected sibs

Sib method corrects for single ascertainment. The corrected segregation ratio is

$$p = (R - N) / (T - N)$$

T = total individuals
R = total affected
N = number of sibships

RACIAL DIFFERENCES

Populations can often be assigned unambiguously to a racial group, but individuals cannot. There are three main types of racial differences:
- anthropometric differences (size, build, colouring, hair type) by which one recognizes (imperfectly) most ethnic groups, but which are not suitable for statistical analysis.
- gene frequencies in polymorphic systems. Blood groups in particular have been studied in vast detail These studies allow indices of genetic distance to be computed between populations and suggest there are three major groupings, Caucasoids, Negroids and Mongoloids.
- individual characters which are especially common or rare in a particular population (Fig. 8.14). The reason may be selection, founder effects or drift. Among blood groups, the Fy allele of the Duffy system, the V antigen of the rhesus

series and the Js^a antigen of the Kell series are markers of Negroid populations.

Genetic drift means the tendency for gene frequencies to change over the generations due to random chance, without selective pressure. Drift is significant only in small populations (populations with 100 or less breeding individuals for a few generations or 1,000 or less for many generations).

Founder effect. If an isolated population stems from a small number of founders, the gene frequencies reflect those in the founders, which by random chance may be different from the source population from which the founders came. Founder effects are a special case of genetic drift.

Character	Comments
dizygotic twinning	high frequency in West Africans
Tay–Sachs disease	common in Ashkenazi Jews
cystic fibrosis	rare in Finland; common in W Europe
phenylketonuria	rare in Finland; common in Ireland
characters associated with resistance to malaria:	
sickle cell disease	West Africa, East Africa
beta thalassaemia	Mediterranean, Middle East
alpha thalassaemia	SE Asia
G6PD deficiency	Mediterranean

Fig. 8.13 Geographically heterogeneous characters.

monozygotic twinning

Down's syndrome and other chromosomal abnormalities

Duchenne muscular dystrophy and other mendelian diseases maintained by recurrent mutation

schizophrenia

Fig. 8.14 Geographically uniform characters.